THE
ALTERNATIVE
MEDICINE
HANDBOOK

THE
ALTERNATIVE
MEDICINE
HANDBOOK

The Complete Reference Guide to
Alternative and Complementary
Therapies

Barrie R. Cassileth, Ph.D.

W. W. NORTON & COMPANY

New York London

FIGURE CREDITS

Alphia Abdikeeva: 4, 31; Lisa B. Cassileth, M.D.: 5, 12, 17, 19, 22, 23, herb drawings in Chapter 11; National Museum of Denmark: 2; Naturhistorisches Museum Wein: 1; Benjamin Ousley: 3, 14, 15, 16, 18, 21, 25, 29, 30; Guenter Rose, Ph.D.: 34; Ross Taylor: 7, 9, 11, 20, 26–28, 32, 33, 35; H. Taylor Vaden: 6, 8, 10, 13, 24.

For information about permission to reproduce selections from this book, write to Permissions, W. W. Norton & Company, Inc., 500 Fifth Avenue, New York, NY 10110.

The text of this book is composed in 10/13 ITC Veljovic Book
with the display set in Charlemagne
Manufacturing by The Haddon Craftsmen, Inc.
Book design and desktop composition by Charlotte Staub.

Library of Congress Cataloging-in-Publication Data

Cassileth, Barrie R.
    The alternative medicine handbook : the complete reference guide to
  alternative and complementary therapies / Barrie R. Cassileth.
      p. cm.
    Includes index.
  ISBN 0-393-04566-8
    1. Alternative medicine—Handbooks, manuals, etc. I. Title.
  R733.C375 1998
  615.5—dc21   97-16268   CIP

W. W. Norton & Company, Inc., 500 Fifth Avenue, New York, N.Y. 10110
http://www.wwnorton.com

W. W. Norton & Company Ltd., 10 Coptic Street, London WC1A 1PU

1 2 3 4 5 6 7 8 9 0

To HTV,
for his patience,
his understanding,
and his support.

CONTENTS

ACKNOWLEDGMENTS

The cancer patients I worked with in the late 1970s introduced me to alternative and complementary therapies. Although these patients were receiving treatment at a major comprehensive cancer center, they simultaneously sought other, unconventional methods. They shared with me their hopes that these "outside" therapies might bring about cures or at least make them feel better. They also shared their concerns over their lack of knowledge about unconventional treatments, whether the treatments worked, and whether they were safe. (Patients and health professionals still ask me these same questions.)

Thus began my research into alternative and complementary therapies, research that produced many professional publications and hopefully information that patients and families found useful. This book is a culmination of those many years of effort and, in part, my way of thanking patients for all that I learned from them.

Unintentionally, this book turned out to be a family project. First came general interest and encouragement. Then my daughter Wendy Junger began sending me relevant news items and publications from California; my other daughter Jodi Greenspan, the young mother of three children, started reporting the use of complementary medicine among her peers; and my daughter-in-law Lisa Cassileth, M.D., now studying to become a surgeon, offered to do some illustrations. Thus my family became not only a very important cheering section, but a source of real and expert help as well. My son Gregory was a superb critic in reviewing chapters, and he contributed greatly to the book's language and content.

There were others who were important to this project. Christopher Chapman and Kim Morgan in Chapel Hill, North Carolina, were able research assistants. I relied importantly on Gerald F. Humphreys, a doctor of divinity (D.Div) and a health services professional, who readily and repeatedly shared information and wise counsel. Sharon Friedman encouraged my desire to produce this book and introduced me to W. W. Norton, where editor Amy Cherry's insight and creative expertise, and Susan Middleton's meticulous copyediting, guided this manuscript toward a more coherent and polished result.

Most of all, I appreciate the help and support of my husband, H. Taylor (Bud) Vaden, who has spent much of his professional life in the health-care field. His continual encouragement and constructive criticism helped make this book what I wanted it to be.

THE
ALTERNATIVE
MEDICINE
HANDBOOK

INTRODUCTION

Most of us grew up depending on mainstream medical care provided by M.D.s who were trained in university-affiliated medical schools. Now many other health resources are available in the form of **alternative** and **complementary** therapies, provided not only by M.D. physicians, but also by other health-care professionals with different initials after their names and different training backgrounds.

What are these new medical alternatives? What do we really know about these methods? Are they safe? Which ones help, and for what problems? Amid the claims and promises, the differences can be difficult to determine. This book will help guide the way by identifying major complementary and alternative medical practices and by describing their backgrounds, goals, benefits, and risks. It neither promotes nor opposes. Rather, it provides clear, impartial information about each method, so that you can make educated health-care decisions.

Some discussion of terminology is helpful at this point. Both terms—*alternative* in the United States and *complementary* in Europe and elsewhere—encompass a wide array of treatments and products. They range from unproven therapies for major illnesses promoted for use in place of mainstream care, to regimens that helpfully accompany mainstream treatment or are used as part of wellness programs. This terminology is unfortunate in that it masks crucial differences among very varied approaches: some therapies are good, helpful, and non-invasive; some are unproven and harmful; others are useless time and money wasters; still others are foolish and fraudulent.

This book treats them differently: **alternative** is

applied to therapies recommended by their practitioners for use *instead of mainstream care* (and thus truly alternative to conventional medicine), while **complementary** is used for therapies that, as the term literally implies, serve a *supplementary role*. Some tend to be promoted primarily as one or the other; others can be either alternative or complementary, depending on how they are used. Aromatherapy is an example. As a soothing fragrance in the bath or during massage, aromatherapy can be pleasant and calming. However, some books and proponents claim that aromatherapy can cure disease, and its use for that alternative purpose could be harmful by delaying needed conventional treatment. Thus, how and when a remedy is applied, as much as what the remedy is, helps to categorize it as appropriate or potentially dangerous.

Alternative therapies tend to be unproven—if their benefits were proven, they are less likely to be considered "alternative." Unproven remedies, such as homeopathy applied for short-term, self-limiting problems, may not be harmful in and of themselves. As with aromatherapy, such therapies can become dangerous if used in lieu of mainstream medical care for serious illnesses.

Complementary therapies—those used alongside medical treatment or as part of a wellness lifestyle—represent a very different group of methods. They are generally noninvasive and helpful, pleasant and stress-reducing, and applicable during sickness and in health.

This book is a road map to help distinguish between empty promises and solid therapies.

In the past, before their causes were discovered, tuberculosis (TB), syphilis, schizophrenia, diabetes, and many other disorders were attributed to emotional problems. A recent example is gastric ulcers. Long believed to be the product of stress, most gastric ulcers are now known to be caused by bacteria. Many cancers represent another current example. Although some practitioners have claimed for years that cancer is caused by stress or personality style, science has recently discovered inherited genetic mutations that cause many types of cancer. For example, a Netherlands study of 9,705 women definitively confirmed other solid research in showing that psychological traits do not play a role in breast cancer risk. Conversely, other recent research suggests that emotional states are much more likely to influence the development of heart disease. Depression and anger, in particular, appear to predict and no doubt contribute to the development of coronary disease.

Overall, these and many other research results tell us that, despite the closeness of the mind-body relationship, we do not always have the ability to intervene. We may be able to neutralize negative emotional states, but we cannot alter inherited genetic mutations no matter how hard we may try to think them away. We can alter behavior to help prevent some illnesses. (For example, 50 percent of cancers are self-induced through behaviors such as smoking and fat-filled diets.) We can adopt lifestyles that maximize health and well-being. We can reach for complementary therapies, self-help techniques, and the best of modern medical technology to help us when serious illness strikes. But we can neither prevent nor cure all ailments, no matter how much we want to and despite the claims of those who sell false hopes in a bottle.

Alternative and complementary therapies are used primarily to maintain health and well-being or to treat minor ailments that will go away themselves in a week or so if left untreated. Many if not most complementary therapies have a powerful ability to reduce stress, which in turn helps ward off many illnesses or reduce their duration or seriousness. The great majority of people who use unconventional remedies when they are seriously ill also receive simultaneous mainstream medical care.

How commonly used are alternative and complementary therapies? It depends on how the terms are defined. If we include Weight Watchers, Alcoholics Anonymous, tea to relieve sore throat, your grandmother's headache remedy, and other self-help, lifestyle activities in addition to therapeutic interventions, alternative and complementary therapies are common indeed. Products or services provided by therapists who claim to treat serious diseases, however, have many fewer adherents. Research shows that alternative and complementary therapies are used most often in the United States to treat anxiety (which is also the most common reason for outpatient visits to mainstream physicians), headaches, and back pain.

Why do people use unconventional medicine? Many explanations have been offered for their great popularity today. One is that self-care, always commonly practiced (most people everywhere have taken care of minor problems themselves), is more highly valued and desired for an even broader range of ailments than in the past. Moreover, appropriate self-care is now encouraged or required by health maintenance organizations (HMOs) or by the high cost of out-of-pocket payments.

The mysticism and ancient beginnings of many unconventional healing practices, such as Ayurveda, traditional Chinese medicine, crystal healing, and others, represent a powerful attraction. There is comfort in using traditions and practices that have flourished since the beginning of history. We become an instant part of honored traditions by adopting their practices and participating in their rituals.

Alternative and complementary approaches often involve belief in a universal energy system. Illness is defined as being out of balance with that spiritual force. Healing involves focusing or rechanneling one's energy, and health is said to occur when the individual is in balance both internally—body, soul, and mind—and with the universe or universal energy. Some people suggest that alternative medicine actually is an alternative religion, and that seeking it fills a kind of spiritual hunger.

My own view is that we have become more interested than ever in the idea of helping ourselves stay healthy and taking control of our well-being, and that we are learning to take advantage of a broader array of preventive and healing techniques. We are drawn to the caring and shared responsibility that typically characterize relationships with practitioners of unconventional medicine. However, most of us are wise enough not to reject the high-tech wonders of mainstream medical care when serious illness strikes, despite conventional medicine's frequent impersonality and its failures to recognize the needs of the patient behind the disease.

Although the basis for much of unconventional medicine is indeed philosophical rather than theoretical or scientific, alternative and complementary therapies can and should be evaluated. In fact, one of the few things that the great diversity of alternative and complementary therapies have in common is that they have not undergone scientific review. Some avid proponents maintain that it is unnecessary to study unconventional therapies, that their longevity and popularity provide adequate "proof" of their validity. But how do we really know when a treatment works? We know after it has been scientifically tested and found to be more effective than doing nothing and at least as effective as other therapies. Comparisons are crucial and feasible—and they help tell us whether a therapy can pose a possible danger to our health.

Anecdotal reports are not adequate. They tell us only that a few people did well, but they reveal nothing about how many people took the same treatment and died or failed to get better, or who recovered because of other therapies, or whose illness got better on its own, as most illnesses do.

Research may move some unconventional practices into the medical mainstream, or show that others produce no benefit. Until real evidence is available, read the guidelines concerning what is known as presented in this book, and see a qualified health professional for serious illnesses and for problems that don't go away in a week. Avoid potentially dangerous or worthless remedies. Some treatment claims should sound an immediate alarm: products that promise easy, miracle cures of major illnesses (such as Alzheimer's and cancer) or reversal of problems that cannot be reversed (such as aging); pressure to use the therapy instead of mainstream treatment you are taking now for a serious disease; assertions of a medical establishment conspiracy to withhold the therapy from the public; claims that the therapy is "natural" and therefore better than prescribed medications. ("Natural" does not necessarily mean "safe"! See Chapter 11.)

Happily, the burgeoning interest in alternative and complementary therapies has been accompanied by a growing interest in studying them properly. There may be unusual aspects to research in this area, but these need not reduce the quality of research required. It is not necessary, for example, to prove or disprove the existence of "prana" or "chi" or any universal energy force in order to study the effect of attempts to manipulate it; nor is it necessary to understand the precise biological action of a remedy to determine whether it relieves pain. Solid research is virtually always possible, and in my view it is always necessary. We need and have a right to know whether healing methods, conventional as well as unconventional, fulfill their proponents' promises.

Research in mainstream medicine is ongoing and well supported by foundations, organizations, corporate sponsors, and most prominently the National Institutes of Health (NIH) in the United States and other countries. Although studies of alternative and complementary medicine were funded by almost all of the eighteen institutes at the NIH for many years before unconventional therapies attained their current popularity, there had been no systematic research effort into their efficacy.

This deficiency was remedied in 1992 with the establishment of the NIH Office of Alternative Medicine. Its purpose is to evaluate alternative and complementary therapies. The creation of such a body in our premier research environment signals the importance of studying unconventional remedies.

This book does not recommend treatments. It describes unconventional techniques, their backgrounds and claims, and provides available evidence about their safety and utility. Fifty-three of the most popular, enduring, and important unconventional therapies or types of therapies are included. Although it is possible to classify unconventional remedies in a number of ways, I have generally used the categories devised by the Office of Alternative Medicine.

This book is divided into seven sections based on that classification. Each section addresses a major type of alternative or complementary treatment: (1) traditional healing methods, which are typically ancient approaches that offer remedies in the context of spiritual and lifestyle guidance; (2) dietary and herbal remedies; (3) methods that involve active use of the mind to heal the body; (4) biologic therapies, which apply unproved pharmacologic and other types of medication; (5) bodywork, involving manipulation of muscles and bones; (6) use of the senses to enhance well-being; and (7) the application of external energy of several types to restore health.

Each section contains several chapters arranged alphabetically. Each chapter includes a brief introduction, followed by a description of the alternative or complementary therapy, claims of practitioners, and the theories or beliefs on which the therapy is based. Then, I describe available research (if any) and what the therapy can do for you. Each chapter ends with a discussion of resources and sources of information. **Boldfaced** type indicates the first occurrence of a defined term, includding concepts cross-referenced to other chapters. A term that is the subject of its chapter is not boldfaced.

I have tried to cut to the core of information that will be most useful, objective, and helpful, and to provide enough insight into alternative and complementary therapies to help guide your decisions. It is important to tell your physician when you are using or planning to try an alternative or complementary remedy, and just as important to become informed and help take charge of your own health and well-being. I hope this book will become your guide.

The information in this book is not a substitute for consultation with your physician. Herbal and other ingested remedies should be discussed first with your health-care professional. This is especially important if you are taking prescription medication.

PART ONE

ROUTES
TO HEALTH
AND SPIRITUAL
FULFILLMENT

The alternative approaches reviewed in this part share many features. Instead of disease-oriented therapies, these are general routes to the maintenance and restoration of health and well-being. They involve much more than prescriptions for ailments. They provide a level of guidance that some see as a substitute for religion. Indeed, most of these alternatives once were or still are thoroughly entwined with religion. And most have endured for hundreds or thousands of years.

In that distant past, medicine, magic, and religion were one and the same. Their combined nature is illustrated in the ancient fertility figures found across Europe. The 30,000-year-old Venus of Willendorf is one of the earliest existing examples (Figure 1). These Venus figures were magical aids to ensure safe births, used to encourage fertility during the time when humans still roamed the earth in search of food. No doubt the great shamans of that time, like those to follow, were both priest and physician, with the extra ability to contact and influence the supernatural forces believed to control all events, including the health of humankind.

The healing systems discussed here originated long before the time of scientific understanding of the human body and its biological mechanisms. It is not surprising, therefore, that both physical and cosmological concerns and uncertainties are reflected in these early explanations of health and illness—not only how the body works and how it changes when death occurs, but also the meaning of celestial events and the relationships among humans, the

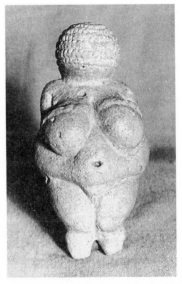

Figure 1 The Venus of Willendorf is one of many small fertility icons found around the world, dating back as far as 30,000 years, during the time when religion, magic, and medicine were combined as one.

environment, the spirit world, and the cosmos.

One of the central ideas shared by these approaches, common to most early efforts to understand health, illness, death, and the human relationship with the larger world, is the notion of an invisible vital energy or life force. Called **prana** in Ayurvedic medicine, **qi** (or *chi*, both pronounced "chee") in traditional Chinese medicine, and by many other terms, the circulation of this vital force could explain life and death. The idea also provided a way of understanding links and pathways between the human body, humankind, the spirit world, and the universe.

It is possible that ancient efforts to improve the flow of human vital energy lie behind peculiar archaeological finds in Europe and South America. Many human skulls dating back to 2000 to 10,000 B.C. have been found with a round plug of bone removed (Figure 2). Healed edges around the hole indicate that at least some people survived the procedure.

Is this procedure, called **trepanation**, evidence of prehistoric cults of healing? The precise rationale for this primitive surgical effort is unknown. Experts believe it was performed as a religious rite, as a way to create an opening for the escape of magical demons, as a treatment to excise bone splinters, or some combination of these. Perhaps it was a means of

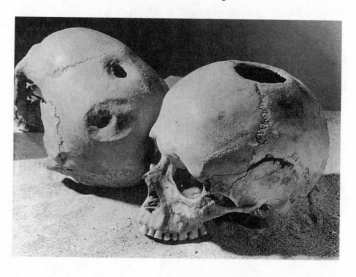

Figure 2 The holes found in ancient, trepanned skulls may be evidence of prehistoric religious or healing rites.

The Alternative Medicine Handbook

improving the flow of human vital energy and bridging the connection between spiritual forces and the mind and body, or a means of draining excess energy. These combined purposes express the unity of religion, magic, and medicine that existed in earliest times.

Another feature common to early healing approaches is efforts to explain physiological events in terms of well-known contrasting pairs: hot–cold, wet–dry, light–dark, active–passive. These qualities were ascribed not only to all bodily components and functions, but also to emotional states, climate, and seasons, achieving the necessary integration of human, space, and time. Early humans made similar connections between body and mind, society and landscape, which all interrelated and reflected one another in a complex system of parallel associations.

Numbers, too, were important and used commonly across the various early healing systems. They provided a means of reflecting universal patterns, controlling human fate, and connecting the activities of the human body with nature's rhythms and cycles. The numbers 4 and 5 predominated as magical in the ancient world. Examples of the latter include the five elements of ancient China, the five elements of the Ayurvedic worldview, the five world regions of pre-Columbian Mexico, and the five senses of Tibetan medicine. The broad significance of the number 4 is evident in descriptions of living creatures and plants, time, elements, ceremonial activity, and points of the sacred hoop in Native American artifacts; it also is found in the ancient Greek conception of bodily humors and the basic elements in the universe.

The healing systems discussed here are not the only or even the earliest such systems. They were selected because they are followed by many people today. Each offers guidance in caring for the body, the mind, and the spirit in an integrated fashion that seems to meet not only the need for physical healing but also fulfills a spiritual hunger as present today as in centuries and millennia past.

1 ⌇

Acupuncture

Although acupuncture is only one component of traditional Chinese medicine, it is a major component and so deserves its own chapter. Acupuncture is a distinct entity because it has its own traditions and conceptual basis, as well as an elaborate system of understanding how the body works. It also has achieved unprecedented widespread acceptance.

One of the most studied of alternative therapies, acupuncture is accepted by mainstream medicine for the management of various types of pain and for addiction control. For this reason, acupuncture is a good example of the few treatments discussed in this book that sit on the cusp between mainstream and alternative medicine: used almost routinely in many conventional hospitals and clinics for certain indications, it is considered alternative or useless as a treatment for other purposes. This treatment technique was popular in ancient China, banned in 1822 by the Chinese Imperial Medical College, which prohibited disrobing as indecent, and rediscovered in the twentieth century. Today, herbal remedies (see Chapter 11) and other traditional techniques (see Chapters 20 and 40) join acupuncture as central components of traditional Chinese medicine.

What It Is

Acupuncture is a medical therapy developed in China more than two thousand years ago. It involves the placement of hair-thin, disposable needles of varying lengths into the skin (Figure 3). Ancient acupuncture needles were made of bone, stone, or metal including silver and gold. Modern needles are made of stainless steel. The needles penetrate just deep enough into the skin to keep from falling out, and skilled practitioners accomplish virtually painless insertion.

Needles are placed at specific points along meridians, or channels. These channels are like rivers with tributaries that flow into increasingly narrow rivulets, mimicking nature's flow of water to increasingly smaller streams. The twelve main meridians, like the twelve main rivers of ancient China, represent an internal sys-

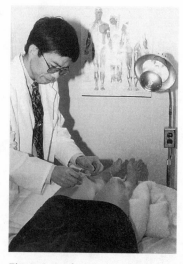

Figure 3 A physician-acupuncturist inserts hair-thin needles into his client.

tem of communication and transport, just as actual waterways permit communication and transport in the outer world. The human body is viewed as a miniature model, or microcosm, of the universe.

Each channel is believed to be connected to a specific networked area or organ system of the body. By needling acupoints along a particular meridian, a problem in a distant area of the body can be treated. (**Acupoints** are points used in both acupuncture and acupressure; see Chapter 32.) In modern acupuncture, more than 1,000 acupoints (some experts say more than 2,000) are recognized, but most treatments require needles in only ten or twelve points. Typically, needles are kept in place for less than one-half hour. Determining the exact size and placement of the needles is essential. Twirling or otherwise setting them into motion is thought to enhance the result.

In classic Chinese medicine, it was believed that every problem, weakness, illness, and symptom could be corrected by acupuncture. Further, this ancient healing method was but one integral piece of a complex mosaic that explained health, disease, the cosmos, and the relationship of humankind with nature and the universe as a whole. This can be seen in the relationship between the number of months and days in a year, and the human body's twelve main meridians, and in the original classic texts the 365 acupoints. The individual pulsates to the rhythm of the cosmos.

Sometimes acupuncture is augmented by **moxibustion**, the placement of a smoldering plug of the herb mugwort on a meridian acupoint. This practice is as old as acupuncture. **Cupping** is another ancient Chinese and Indian remedy in which heated cups are placed on the skin, sometimes after small punctures are made at the intended location. This process produces a suction force that is thought to boost circulation and improve health.

A variation of acupuncture—deep finger pressure on acupoints—is known as **acupressure**. It is similar to Japanese shiatsu. Insertion of acupuncture needles only in the outer ear is a relatively new variation in which the ear serves as a miniature map of the entire body and its acupoints.

A Cure for All Problems

Originally, acupuncture was used to treat all ailments by restoring balance within the individual, and between the individual and the universe.

Modern Acupuncture

Modern versions of acupuncture use electricity, heat, laser beams, sonar rays, and other nonneedle acupoint stimulators.

In use since the 1930s, electroacupuncture is considered less tiring and time-consuming than the manual version. Needles are connected to a supply of weak electric power. Therapeutic reactions are said to be just as effective.

What Practitioners Say It Does

In China, acupuncture is still applied to treat ailments and cure disease, although research does not support its ability to cure. Acupuncture is applied, for example, to correct the abnormal fetal positions of unborn babies, cardiac problems, and gynecologic disorders, among other problems. Overall, results across studies in each of these areas are disappointing, and carefully conducted investigations find no benefit. The National Institutes of Health recently began a $2.5 million study to look at the effects of acupuncture on asthma.

In modern Chinese hospitals, acupuncture sometimes is used as a secondary surgical anesthetic. In the West, acupuncture is used primarily to relieve pain and other symptoms such as nausea and vomiting, and to assist withdrawal from addictions such as drug and alcohol dependency. Research does support its effectiveness for these purposes.

Beliefs on Which It Is Based

Classic, traditional acupuncture is based on ancient Chinese medicine and its understanding of health. The origins of acupuncture illustrate how the earliest civilizations sought to understand the world and its various components, including seasons, nature, wellness, and disease, as parts of a single whole. Each aspect of life, including health and disease, was conceptualized as a polarity, manipulated by two opposing forces in nature. These forces are the **yin**, or dark female force, and the **yang**, or light male force. Illness was said to occur when opposing yin-yang energies were not in harmony. Acupuncture and all other healing interventions, such as herbal tonics or *qigong*, aimed to rebalance these energies.

This deceptively simple idea is actually an extremely complex, detailed set of interactions and connections among bodily organs, forces, and pathways. A central component of the belief system is the idea of vital energy, or the life force. In classic Chinese medicine, the life force is termed *chi* or *ch'i*, or in modern transliteration *qi* (all pronounced "chee").

When there is a balance of *qi*—not too much or too little flow of energy—there is good health. An excess or

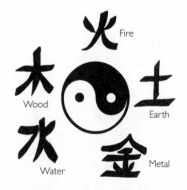

Figure 4 The Chinese names for the five elements (fire, earth, metal, water, and wood) are shown here surrounding the traditional Chinese yin-yang symbol.

deficiency in the flow of energy, however, represents an imbalance that causes pain and illness. Acupuncture is applied to correct that imbalance. An uneven flow of *qi* is returned to equilibrium by the placement of acupuncture needles along or at the intersections of appropriate meridians.

The twelve main meridians traverse the body and culminate in the toes or fingertips. They connect the exterior environment to the interior of the body and link the internal organs to one another and thus to the outer world. Each of the individual meridians relates to a particular organ and is called by that organ's name (for example, the gall bladder meridian). The system is made more exact and increasingly complex with the addition of yet other factors, primarily the natures of the affected meridians and organs, plus a subtle, social and moral notion of each person's relationship to the broader harmony of nature, the seasons, and the universe.

Classic Chinese medicine describes six "solid," or yin, organs, such as heart and lungs, and six "hollow," or yang, organs, including stomach and intestine. Each organ is perceived to be under the control of one of the five elements, or manifestations of *qi*, of which all matter was thought to be composed: water, fire, wood, metal, and earth (Figure 4). (Later, in the sixth century B.C., a similar idea using four rather than five basic "humors"—water, fire, earth, and air—was adopted in Greece.)

Each organ, tied to the universe through its dominat-

Examples of the Twelve Meridians

(Energy pathways along which *qi* circulates throughout the body. Many acupoints dot each meridian.)

The Gallbladder Meridian starts at the eye, runs back and forth across the skull, goes down the shoulders, and then descends by the side of the body until it ends in the fourth toe. A yang meridian, its function is balanced by its yin counterpart, the liver meridian.

The Spleen Meridian runs from the armpit through the chest and abdomen, across the hip and down the leg to its conclusion in a toe. Twenty-one acupoints dot its length.

---

ing life-force element, was also associated with the person's feelings, thoughts, and behavior. Emotions, it was believed, dwelt in and pertained to specific organs: sorrow lived in the lungs, happiness dwelt in the heart, the soul and anger both resided in the liver. Lecherous ideas led to diseases of the lung; acting on such ideas caused heart problems, and so on. To effect a cure, the healer had to determine the objectionable behavior and the mental state that changed the organ and caused the illness. When the origin of disharmony was detected, a remedy in the form of particular acupoints was designed.

Research Evidence to Date

Acupuncture does work well to relieve the pain of arthritis, PMS, and other chronic pain, and to ease withdrawal symptoms associated with alcoholism, drug addiction, and smoking. Just how it works remains unknown, and the existence of meridians also remains unproven. The fundamental idea of a vital life force that can become unbalanced and rechanneled as it courses through the body remains an ancient concept in which many continue to believe. However, there is no scientific evidence that supports its existence.

While some investigators continue to search for proof of meridians and vital life energy, others study additional claims. Acupuncture's ability to relieve disorders or symptoms such as osteoporosis, migraine, and sinusitis, for example, awaits scientific proof.

Acupuncture does not, however, cure disease. It is applied today for that purpose primarily in underdeveloped areas of Asia where access to modern medicine is unavailable.

What It Can Do for You

If you have unexplained symptoms or a serious medical illness, see a conventional physician and take advantage of modern diagnostic and treatment techniques. These can catch a serious problem early when it is most treatable, rule out the existence of a serious problem, or provide the best chance of cure. Acupuncture is not a realistic alternative to modern diagnostic or therapeutic techniques.

However, if your sore knee still leaves you limping or your pain persists, acupuncture might well be your best bet. Its simplicity, lack of toxicity or complications, low cost, and frequent effectiveness make acupuncture a therapy of choice for various kinds of chronic pain (when the reason for it has been uncovered and conventional treatment is not preferred). Try it also to help relieve the difficulties of addiction withdrawal, arthritis, headaches, and other problems that have no treatable underlying cause.

Some people use acupuncture to decrease stress, although no research supports the effectiveness of acupuncture for this purpose. If it works for you, it hardly matters that we cannot find *qi* or that skeptics think it is a placebo.

Where to Get It

✦ There are approximately 6,500 acupuncture practitioners in the United States today. In addition to those trained primarily as acupuncturists, more than 3,000 M.D.s and D.O.s (doctors of osteopathy) in the United States have attended courses in acupuncture and incorporate it into their practices. Such training programs are affiliated with major medical centers such as those at the University of California, Los Angeles, and New York University.

✦ Many conventional physicians refer patients to well-trained and experienced acupuncturists.

✦ Qualified acupuncturists may be recommended by one of the national associations that provide names of practitioners who meet competency standards, such as the American Association of Acupuncture and Oriental Medicine in Pennsylvania (610 266-1433), or the National Commission for the Certification of Acupuncturists in Washington, D.C. (202 232-1404).

✦ Licensure and regulations regarding the practice of acupuncture vary across the United States. Legislation in twenty-six states plus the District of Columbia regulate the practice of acupuncture, and sixteen states grant licenses to practice acupuncture. Requirements and regulations differ broadly across states.

The Acupuncture Advantage

· It provides effective relief for many kinds of pain.
· It may help when conventional pain therapies do not.
· Side effects are all but nonexistent.
· It is painless.
· It is inexpensive.

2

Ayurveda

About 1500 B.C., Aryan invaders from the north of what would later become India drove the earlier inhabitants down into the Indian subcontinent. The invaders brought with them their literature, hymns, prayers, teachings, and manuscripts. This body of knowledge and literature was known as the Vedas—Sanskrit for "knowledge"—and it formed the basis for the subsequent development of India's moral, religious, cultural, and medical codes. Thus, Ayurvedic ("knowledge of life") medicine sprang from the information in the Vedas, expanded by many later commentaries and additional medical writings. As its English translation suggests, Ayurveda encompasses religion and philosophy as well as medicine and science.

What It Is

Ayurvedic medicine is one of the few ancient healing systems that remains popular today, although in greatly modified and modernized form. It is based on the idea that illness is the absence of physical, emotional, and spiritual harmony. Thus it stresses proper physical and mental self-care to ensure good health and enhance longevity. Ayurvedic medicine, therefore, encompasses prevention and health maintenance as well as diagnosis and treatment.

Many of Ayurveda's basic principles are similar to those of Chinese medicine. Both involve concepts such as life force (the energy that sustains life); balance; the integral relationship among body, mind, environment, and nature; the importance of tongue and pulse evaluation for diagnosing illness; and breathing exercises. India's medical methodologies influenced and helped shape important aspects of Chinese healing systems.

Ayurveda, as well as other ancient systems of belief and healing, often appear strange, primitive, or irrational to those raised in modern societies where understanding the body and the world rests on scientific proof. Ancient healing systems tend to remain essentially unchanged across millennia, in contrast to modern science and medicine, which continually grow and change through constant questioning, evolution, and proof. According to contemporary experts, Ayurvedic science is based not on constantly emerging research data but on the eternal wisdom of those who received this cosmic consciousness through religious introspection and meditation.

Today's Ayurvedic practitioners claim to bring about well-being, the prevention of disease, and the harmony of body and mind by aligning patients' lifestyles with their individual constitutions and personal medical histories. The primary tools of Ayurvedic medicine include maintaining certain lifestyle habits such as diet; using natural medicines, herbs, and internal cleansing preparations; and doing various yoga and meditation exercises. Ayurvedic visual images, as seen in ancient paintings and sculpture, convey the peace and balance that Ayurveda strives to attain.

What Practitioners Say It Does

The main goal of Ayurvedic therapies is to restore the body's **homeostasis**, or the balance of one's metabolic forces. This is accomplished by applying or following Ayurvedic treatments, including breathing exercises, diets, physical activity, herbal tonics, elimination therapies and other purification procedures, meditation, and massage. Each therapy is personalized according to the individual's problems and metabolic characteristics. These programs are said to maintain health and prevent disease, enhance mental health, and treat illness.

In the last few decades, a modernized, commercial version of Ayurvedic healing has emerged. Promoters offer lectures, books, audio programs, and other self-help instructional materials based on traditional Ayurvedic healing. Transcendental Meditation is emphasized.

This modern movement is viewed by many with concern. Published testimonials expressing profound dissatisfaction as well as sites on the World Wide Web maintained by the Cult Awareness Network deal with the shortcomings, dissatisfactions, and risks of the program marketed as Transcendental Meditation. Meditation is an essential component of Ayurvedic culture. The trademarked Transcendental Meditation, conversely, is largely a commercial enterprise that claims many benefits for its members and for society. However, some authorities believe the TM movement is drawing young people into a private and exploitative world of potential harm.

Beliefs on Which It Is Based

Under one complex and encompassing concept, Ayurveda describes an understanding of people and of the cosmos in which everything is interrelated and interdependent. Practitioners believe that there are three **doshas**, or basic metabolic types (*Kapha, Pitta,* and *Vata*). Each is located in specific body organs, and each is associated with two of Ayurveda's five environmental elements (earth, water, fire, air, and ether). In Ayurveda, each element corresponds to one of the five senses, as well as to areas of the body. It is believed that ether is related to hearing and to open spaces in the mind, air to touch, fire to sight, water to taste, and earth to smell. Color, emotions, seasons, and time of day all are seen as interrelated, as Figure 5 shows.

Doshas are the bridging force among organs and internal parts of the body. They also connect the body with environmental or cosmic elements. Although each person is believed to be a combination of characteristics

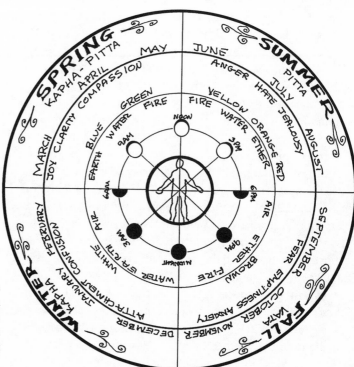

Figure 5 This mandala shows the relationship between human characteristics, seasons, the elements, and the cosmos in ancient Ayurvedic teaching

	KAPHA	**PITTA**	**VATA**
Physical characteristics and style	Heavy; pale, oily skin; thick hair; slow-moving; relaxed	Ruddy skin; fair hair; medium build; loving; compulsive	Slender; cool skin; nervous; energetic; intuitive
Metabolic characteristics	Prone to obesity, high cholesterol, and allergies	Prone to heartburn, ulcers, hemorrhoids, and acne	Prone to nervous disorders, anxiety, constipation, and moods
Internal organ location	Lungs; chest; spinal fluid	Stomach; blood; small intestine; skin; eyes	Large intestine; pelvic cavity; bones; ears
Associated natural elements	Water and earth	Fire and water	Air and ether
Physiological role	Nourishes, protects, and stabilizes body	Digestion; metabolism *Kapha-Vata* interface	Movement; breathing; blood circulation

from all three *doshas*, one *dosha* type predominates in each person. The predominant *dosha* describes the individual's physical, metabolic, and emotional characteristics, as well as his or her daily habits and lifestyle.

In addition to defining predominant body types, characteristics, and appearances, *doshas* provide other vital functions. Their metabolic role is to keep the body intact and functional. They also maintain a balance among internal body organs. It is believed that all bodily functions are under *dosha* control. The *doshas*, their characteristics, and associations are given in the accompanying chart.

Maintaining and restoring good health requires bringing the three *doshas* back into balance. This process involves and is aided by reducing emotional stress, improving one's lifestyle, and ridding the body of accumulated toxins. Diet and therapies are prescribed on the basis of the individual's predominant *dosha* type.

Ayurvedic diagnostic techniques employ three main activities: inspection, palpation, and questioning. It is important to observe the tongue, nails, and lips, plus each of the body's nine "doors" (two eyes, two ears, two nostrils, mouth, genitalia, and anus) and their secretions. Tapping and listening to the lungs, feeling other parts of the body, and taking the pulse reveal strengths as well as weaknesses. Taking the history includes learning details about the life and health of the patient—past, present, and intended future.

As in Chinese medicine, the Ayurvedic system of pulse taking is extremely detailed and much more time-

Chakras

Traversing the body from the base of the spine to the head, seven **chakras,** or energy centers, are believed to link to internal organs, natural elements, colors, and deities. Self-illumination is said to occur when energy reaches the topmost chakra.

consuming than in Western medicine. Diagnoses are described in terms of organ system imbalances, which in turn are tied to imbalances of the *doshas*. The goal of treatment is to restore *dosha* balance.

Therapies address diet and lifestyle. Dietary treatments include recommendations and cautions against foods for particular *doshas*. Specific foods are thought to weaken or strengthen *doshas*. Lifestyles choices concerning waking, eating, sleeping times, and sexual habits are recommended for particular *doshas* or to correct *dosha* imbalances. Medicinals include herbs, spices, metals, or other natural products that are believed to be related or tied to specific ailments, body types, or imbalances. Breathing exercises and yoga also are recommended, again according to ailments and *dosha* type.

Another aspect of traditional Ayurvedic treatment is its focus on removing toxins from the body, which occurs after diagnosis and before other treatments are begun. In India as in North America, this purging is still accomplished according to ancient practice. These methods, known as *panchakarma,* include bloodletting (typically by applying leeches), induced vomiting, and bowel purging.

It is of interest to note that in India today, traditional Ayurvedic medicine has been institutionally modified to incorporate many Western practices. A survey revealed that 75 percent of drugs used by Indian Ayurvedic doctors were modern medications such as antibiotics. Ayurvedic practitioners are now analyzing the properties of herbs prescribed in the ancient texts by electron microscopy and computers. Ironically, it is the older Ayurvedic practices, such as using leeches and other unattractive components typically discarded by the modernized Ayurveda, toward which people in the United States gravitate.

Research Evidence to Date

Many Ayurvedic practitioners believe that regimens based on *doshas* can be used to diagnose and treat virtually all disorders, including serious illnesses. However, there is no scientific evidence that they work for such purposes. If you have or may have a serious disease, Ayurvedic healing techniques should not be relied on to cure the illness.

Meditation, an important component of today's popular Ayurvedic medicine, has been subjected to research over the years. Meditation has been shown to reduce anxiety, help lower hypertension, and enhance general well-being. There is as yet no scientific research that documents the ability of herbs or other components of the Ayurvedic system to cure disease, but studies of the potential benefits of Ayurvedic herbal compounds continue.

What It Can Do for You

Most people turn to Ayurvedic techniques for the sense of rejuvenation, harmony, and calm that they inspire. Meditation can slow the pulse and relax the mind. Its calming effects can be very useful, and many people meditate as part of a regular health maintenance regimen.

Ayurvedic's emphasis on self-care is consistent with today's emphasis on personal responsibility for one's health. Healthy or ill, many achieve the serenity and sense of well-being that these ancient techniques can bring. Furthermore, engaging in healing practices that predate current understanding of human physiology may have benefits in and of itself. Many enjoy the idea that their herbal teas or meditation practices were in use thousands of years ago.

Where to Get It

There is no program of licensure for Ayurvedic practitioners in the United States. Those who practice Ayurvedic medicine may be physicians, chiropractors, nutritionists, or other healers. The best and most responsible Ayurvedic practitioners encourage clients with serious illnesses to see conventional physicians also.

✦ The Ayurvedic Institute in Albuquerque, New Mexico (505 291-9698), provides training in various aspects of Ayurveda.

✦ Some elements of Ayurvedic healing, such as meditation or massage, are available from practitioners who specialize in these particular methods. Usually such practitioners can be found in telephone directories.

✦ Libraries, health-food stores, and bookshops have information and self-help guides to Ayurvedic practices.

Attraction of Ayurveda

There is comfort in sharing experiences that are thousands of years old.

Identification with ancestral roots, engaging in activities used by those who shared this earth and sky long ago, and the sense of cosmic community are all part of Ayurvedic healing.

3

Chinese Medicine, Traditional

Lao-tzu, the sixth-century B.C. founder of Taoism, laid the groundwork for traditional Chinese medicine. He described the necessary balance of opposite and complementary forces termed yin and yang, explained the disorder and illness that result from any imbalance of these internal and universal forces, and described the important role of *qi* (pronounced "chee," and sometimes written *chi* or *ch'i*), the vital energy force that flows through the body.

President Nixon was accompanied on his groundbreaking visit to China in 1972 by many reporters, among them James Reston, a highly-respected writer for the *New York Times*. At one point, Mr. Reston suffered severe pain in his abdomen and was rushed to the Anti-Imperialist Hospital in Beijing. Surgeons removed his appendix using conventional anesthesia. All went well until the following evening, when Mr. Reston suffered further severe abdominal pain. Instead of receiving the usual pain-killing pills, however, he was treated by the hospital acupuncturist who inserted needles into his elbow and below his knees. The pain disappeared immediately and permanently. A few days later, the story of James Reston's medical experience appeared under his byline on the front page of the *New York Times*.

This single account contributed greatly to Americans' awareness of many aspects of Chinese culture, especially the ancient system of treatment with acupuncture. Although Westerners tend to be familiar with acupuncture (see Chapter 1), Chinese medicine encompasses other equally important techniques, and all exist within a comprehensive, alternative system of anatomy, physiology, and healing.

What It Is

Chinese medicine is a complete system of health care that has been in use for almost three millennia. It includes prevention as well as treatments for various disorders. Diagnosis, therapy, terminology, and understanding of the human physiology and how the body works in traditional Chinese medicine are profoundly different from those of Western medicine. Importantly, traditional Chinese medicine has changed relatively little over the centuries. This contrasts with Western medicine, which is constantly in flux, changing as new information and data clarify understanding of health and illness, and as research evaluates the effectiveness of therapies and generates new treatments.

The cornerstone concept in Chinese medicine is *qi*, which is conceptualized as energy that flows through the body along pathways known as meridians. In Chinese medicine, ailments are attributed to an imbalance of *qi*. Diagnostic efforts focus on determining the state of a patient's *qi*, including any excesses or deficiencies. Therapies, all of which aim to balance *qi*, include acupuncture, moxibustion, cupping, massage, herbal remedies, and the practice of meditation, concentration, and exercise known as *qigong*. With the exception of moxibustion and cupping, this book contains chapters discussing each of these therapies, and all are described briefly below.

What Practitioners Say It Does

Unlike Western medicine, Chinese medicine is not disease-specific. It is concerned instead with discovering the unique underlying dysfunction that allows illness to develop in a particular individual. Like Western medicine, traditional Chinese medicine is used to treat a wide variety of ailments with several basic therapeutic tools.

Acupuncture involves the insertion of needles at specific, predetermined points on the body, called acupuncture points or acupoints, which correspond to the meridians through which *qi* is believed to flow throughout the body. Acupuncture is discussed in more detail in Chapter 1.

Moxibustion involves burning a small mound of tightly bound leaves of an herb known as the Chinese mugwort, or *Artemisia vulgaris*. The leaves are burned directly on the body near *qi* meridians associated with the patient's particular ailment, or near places in the body suspected of being deficient in *qi*. The heat generated by moxibustion is believed to penetrate deeply into the body, restoring its internal balance and strengthening its *qi*.

Cupping is similar to moxibustion in that it involves

directing energy to a specific part of the body. Rather than using burning leaves, cupping creates suction above the part of the body that requires treatment. Suction is created by warming the air inside a glass jar and turning the jar over on the patient's body. The vacuum created by the heat is said to dispel dampness from the body, warm the *qi,* and reduce swelling. Cupping is recommended particularly for cases of bronchial congestion and chronic ailments such as arthritis and bronchitis.

Several systems of **massage** are used in traditional Chinese medicine. Two that date back to the Han dynasty (200 B.C.–A.D. 200) are *an-mo* and *tuina.* In *an-mo* the massage therapist uses pressing and rubbing motions on affected areas of the body; in *tuina* a thrusting and rolling type of massage is applied. Chinese massage is practiced on the same points of the body used in acupuncture, and with the same aim: to detect areas of excessive, deficient, or blocked *qi,* to unblock those areas, and to bring *qi* back into balance.

Qigong is a series of activities that involve breathing, exercise, and meditation to balance and strengthen *qi.* *Qigong* literally means "manipulation of vital energy." There are two major forms of *qigong:* internal and external. In internal *qigong,* patients perform exercises of breathing and movement to strengthen their own *qi.* The related system of movement and breathing known as tai chi, popular in China and becoming well known in other countries, uses *qigong* and is considered a type of *qigong* exercise.

Other forms of internal *qigong* exist, each involving meditation and breathing. In fact, there are more than 100 schools of internal *qigong* in China, and well over 3,000 schools have existed historically.

External *qigong* involves the transfer of *qi* from a *qigong* master to the body of another individual. This may be accomplished either by the master touching areas on the other person's body, or indirectly, as the master stands nearby, consciously striving to transmit his energy to the patient. It is said that *qi* masters have developed the art of causing their own energy to flow outside of their bodies to influence the health of others or to move inanimate objects. *Qigong* is detailed in Chapter 20 and tai chi in Chapter 40.

Herbal medicine is an ancient mainstay of traditional Chinese practice. Just as Chinese medicine's view of the body differs significantly from that of Western medicine, so does its system of administering medicine. Most drugs in Chinese medicine are time-honored herbal preparations, part of an herbal formulary developed over the centuries. In addition to its more than 3,000 herbs, the formulary also includes animal and mineral ingredients. Remedies are applied to treat a spectrum of ailments, from self-limiting illnesses and minor pains to major diseases such as cancer.

Herbs and their effects are described using the language of Chinese medicine. That is, they are classified by their effects on *qi*, balance, and the five elements (fire, earth, metal, water, and wood). Often herbal medicines are combined in sophisticated ways not only to cure patients' particular ailments, but also to restore the overall balance of their systems. Herbs usually are administered in combinations, prepared typically by boiling to create an herbal tea. As a patient's condition changes, the mix of herbs prescribed is altered accordingly.

Beliefs on Which It Is Based

In addition to balance and energy, the concept of yin-yang and the idea of five elements are central to traditional Chinese medical understanding. **Yin-yang** refers to the interaction between opposite forces, such as male-female, active-passive, and dark-light. Imbalances of yin and yang are believed to manifest themselves in too much or too little activity in particular body organs. A yin-yang balance throughout the body must be maintained to sustain health.

Closely related to the idea of balance is the system of the five Chinese elements. Each organ and bodily system is associated with one of these elements. The elements are considered to be the essential components of the universe. Therapies are prescribed to correct excesses or deficiencies in these elements. The elements and their corresponding organs are believed to influence each other in predetermined ways. For example, fire comes from wood. Hence the function of an organ associated with fire (the heart) is influenced by an organ associated with wood (the liver).

It should be noted that *qi*, yin and yang, and the system of the five elements have no analogues in Western medicine. They represent an alternative way of thinking about the body and disease.

The system of the five elements is central also to traditional Chinese diagnoses. Practitioners rely heavily on the system of elements as well as on thorough pulse taking. Pulse evaluation involves not just the wrist pulse used by Western doctors, but also other, more detailed readings. Doctors typically take twelve pulses, as each pulse is believed to correspond to a different internal organ. Traditional Chinese doctors also pay close attention to the appearance and condition of the patient's tongue, which is thought to provide clues to underlying disease.

Diagnosis and a treatment plan follow according to the Chinese concept of internal bodily relationships and the entire cosmology of traditional Chinese medicine. A patient diagnosed with pneumonia by a Western doctor, for example, might be given the traditional Chinese diagnosis of deficiency of liver *qi* or excess of heat in the spleen. Treatment would differ according to which of the two dysfunctions, liver or spleen, is perceived to have caused the problem, because the pneumonia is viewed as the outer manifestation of the cause of the illness. In Western medicine, all patients diagnosed with pneumonia would be treated with the same antibiotics, while to a traditional Chinese doctor, patients presenting with pneumonia could be treated with any number of therapies according to what the underlying ailment is determined to be.

Research Evidence to Date

Of the major components of traditional Chinese medicine, some have been well documented by modern research as effective therapeutic techniques. Acupuncture (see Chapter 1) can control chronic pain in many instances, and it often works effectively to help break addictive drug habits. Moxibustion and cupping are still used in Chinese hospitals, but they are used much less frequently in other settings, and they lack the documentation now associated with acupuncture.

Qigong enhances balance and muscle tone, and is

especially useful for people who are frail, such as elderly persons or patients with serious debilitating ailments like cancer. The situation with herbal remedies is more complex, as each of the thousands of herbs contain several parts (root, leaf, stem, flower), and as several herbs typically are combined to produce remedies. Many herbal remedies appear to be safe and effective; some are not.

Because the Food and Drug Administration (FDA) is not required to regulate herbal preparations, manufacturers are not obliged to specify their ingredients. Therefore, consumers cannot know whether a product for sale on a store shelf contains what it says it does, whether it is pure, or whether it includes potentially dangerous elements or contaminants.

Ginseng, among the best-known Asian herbs, is a good example of the promises and problems of herbal medicine. Extolled for its virtues over many centuries, it has not yet been subjected to adequate scientific testing to document the circumstances under which it is effective and safe. Contradictory research has led to its sale to treat opposing symptoms, so that it is marketed both as a stimulant and as a depressant. Further, analyses of fifty-four ginseng products indicated that 25 percent contained no ginseng at all, and 60 percent contained only trace amounts.

As the demand for ginseng and other Chinese herbs has soared, the Chinese government recently issued curbs on the production of traditional herbal medicines, citing the ready availability of adulterated, fake, and illegal remedies. The Chinese Ministry of Health indicated that adulterated medicines, available without a doctor's prescription, are causing disabilities and deaths. China plans to close all substandard factories and markets, as well as those trading in medicines banned by the state. However, because herbal remedies from China are still available in the West, and because American and other producers are not under these controls, be wary of any herbal remedies you wish to purchase.

What It Can Do for You

Many aspects of Chinese medicine enhance well-being and have other important roles in health care. In addition to acupuncture and *qigong,* meditation and massage have been shown to lower anxiety and increase feelings of relaxation. Many herbal remedies show potential promise, but experts caution that better research and the implementation of quality control standards are still necessary.

Where to Get It

The practice and licensing of specialists in Asian (including Chinese) medicine is regulated on a state by state basis in the United States. Most practitioners in the United States specialize in either acupuncture or massage. Many states regulate the practice of acupuncture, but few regulate other aspects of Chinese medicine. California and Nevada require those licensed in acupuncture also to demonstrate knowledge of herbal medicine.

New Mexico has established a profession of "oriental medicine," which both restricts others from practicing it and establishes a scope of activity for licensed practitioners similar to that of primary-care physicians.

Names of local practitioners of Chinese and other Asian medicine may be obtained from:

✦ American Association of Acupuncture and Oriental
   Medicine
   4101 Lake Boone Trail, Suite 201
   Raleigh, NC 27607
   Telephone: (919) 787-5181

Those receiving conventional medical care while seeing a practitioner of Chinese medicine should inform both practitioners, so that treatment may be coordinated and the patient alerted to any interactions or conflicts between the two therapies.

For practitioners, mastering the components of traditional Chinese medicine, such as herbal medicine, requires many years of study and practice. As when evaluating the background of any health-care provider, you should determine the length of training and time in practice of a traditional Chinese medicine practitioner.

Homeopathy

Homeopathy and mainstream medicine approach illness from opposite ends of the problem. Homeopathy starts with the study of cures, while mainstream medicine begins with the study of disease. Mainstream science seeks to destroy the virus or other cause of sickness before the disease has a chance to develop or progress. Conversely, homeopathy begins by looking for cures through the study of symptoms.

Homeopathy was developed by Samuel Hahnemann (Figure 6), a German physician of the late eighteenth century. Rebelling against the harmful and barbarous practices of prescientific medicine of the time, such as bloodletting and purging, he founded a more humane approach based on the use of tiny doses of substances that produced in volunteers the same symptoms experienced by the patient.

The Law of Proving is the homeopathic principle by which substances were evaluated for their healing effect. Hahnemann, his assistants, and followers conducted many provings, ingesting plants, minerals, and other substances and carefully recording the symptoms each substance produced. When future patients displayed similar symptoms, they were treated with extremely diluted doses of that substance. This approach became the first law of homeopathy: the Law of Similars, or "like cures like."

Eventually, volumes of descriptions were collected by Hahnemann and his volunteers. These volumes, called the *Homeopathic Pharmacopoeia,* have been used ever since as the basis for homeopathic remedies. When a patient describes his or her symptoms, they are compared against this huge compendium of documented symptoms until a match is found. The patient is then treated with a highly diluted version of that substance. A person complaining of vomiting and diarrhea, for example, might be treated with an extremely high dilution of a poisonous plant called the thorn apple, because a tiny bite of that plant causes vomiting and diarrhea. This is an example of "like cures like."

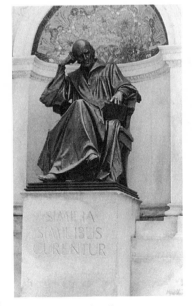

Figure 6 Samuel Hahnemann was the German founder of modern homeopathy. The inscription on his statue in Washington, D.C., is Latin for "like cures like."

What It Is

Homeopathy was one of the original alternatives to conventional modern medicine. While translating the writings of William Cullen, a Scottish professor of medicine, Hahnemann learned of quinine as a possible cure for malaria. Testing the medicine on himself, Hahnemann noticed that tiny amounts of quinine induced the same shaking and fever brought about by the disease itself, and concluded that quinine cures malaria because the drug produces the symptoms of malaria in a healthy person. In actuality, quinine cures malaria by killing the mosquito-borne parasite that causes it.

The idea was that large doses of a substance cause a symptom, while very small doses of that same substance will cure it. During the sixteenth century, a physician named Paracelsus supposedly cured people of the plague by giving them a piece of bread containing a droplet of their own excrement. Hahnemann's rationale was that homeopathic remedies would replace the disease with a similar, but weaker illness that the body's "vital force" could more easily overcome.

What Practitioners Say It Does

Homeopathic remedies typically are applied today to treat chronic and transient conditions such as arthritis, asthma, colds, flu, and allergies, for which the vast majority of patients seek general medical attention. However, some practitioners, many of them not M.D.s, believe that homeopathic remedies can cure any and every illness. Despite the fact that homeopathic remedies cannot substitute for insulin in diabetes or for the surgical removal of a tumor, some proponents claim that homeopathic remedies can cure these as well as other serious, potentially life-threatening diseases.

Responsible practitioners do not use homeopathic remedies to treat diabetes, cancer, or other major illnesses such as heart disease, or to treat surgical emergencies, serious infections, or bad injuries.

Beliefs on Which It Is Based

The word *homeopathy,* coined by Hahnemann, is derived from the Greek words *homoios* ("similar") and *pathos* ("suffering" or "sickness"). This translates roughly to "like cures like," which remains one of the main concepts on which homeopathy is based. Another is the dilution effect: the more dilute the dose, the more powerful the remedy's effect. This use of highly diluted substances persists as homeopathy's most unscientific and problematic aspect.

Homeopathic remedies are made from plants, minerals, animal products, or chemicals diluted many times, usually in water, sometimes in alcohol. Between each subsequent dilution the compound is shaken vigorously, perhaps 100 times. A 1-in-100 dilution, for example, means that one drop of a plant extract is placed in ninety-nine drops of water or alcohol. After vigorous, lengthy shaking, one drop of the new solution is mixed with another ninety-nine drops of water, and the mixture is again shaken vigorously. This procedure may continue twenty, thirty, or more times. In the end, the resulting solution can be more than a billion times more dilute than a solution of one molecule of salt placed in an ocean. Since a molecule is the smallest possible amount of any substance, most homeopathic remedies contain less than one molecule of the original plant or mineral extract. This makes it safe in case your baby swallows an entire bottle, but can it work?

Herein lies the dilemma of homeopathy. If there's nothing in the remedy, how can it affect symptoms or disease?

The explanation most commonly offered by homeopaths is that the remedy's water retains a "trace memory" in the form of electromagnetic frequencies of the active ingredient it once contained. The vigorous shakings between each dilution are thought to activate this chemical memory. Alternately, it is suggested that the process may release the essence, or healing life force, of the original substance.

There are two main difficulties with the "trace memory" hypothesis. The first is that liquids are not known to have memories. The second is that even if liquids could contain trace memories of homeopathic solutions, they also would contain trace memories of all the other substances removed by purification procedures during water recycling, including those that might negate the

A Typical Homeopathic Visit

A patient comes in feeling weak and slightly dizzy. The homeopathic practitioner studies the patient through observation and questioning. The patient has a flushed appearance suggesting fever, rapid heartbeat, and difficulty sleeping.

With this knowledge, the practitioner will locate a substance that produces those same symptoms in a healthy person.

When the patient takes the remedy (a vastly diluted solution of the substance) as prescribed, the symptoms—weakness, fever, rapid heartbeat, and so on—are supposed to disappear promptly.

effects of the original substance or that might have harmful effects of their own.

Research Evidence to Date

Homeopathy's inability to provide an explanation of how its remedies work that can be tested for reproducible results has been a perplexing problem for proponents and a major source of scientific skepticism. Some homeopaths suggest that conventional treatments such as immunization and allergy therapies work as homeopathy is said to work, according to the Law of Similars, and that they both also use small amounts of a substance.

The problem here is that conventional inoculations consist of substances that are identical or similar to disease-causing agents, while homeopathic remedies typically use agents quite different from those that cause disease. In other words, homeopathy relies on the similarity between symptoms provoked by remedies and those caused by the illness, not on the sameness between disease agents and remedies. Furthermore, immunizations do not contain less than one molecule of a substance, and they work directly on the immune response.

Testing Homeopathic Remedies?

In 1938, homeopath and U.S. Senator Royal Copeland of New York included a special release for homeopathic remedies in the Federal Food, Drug, and Cosmetic Act. This act later came under the aegis of the Food and Drug Administration (FDA).

The provision exempted all substances listed in the *Homeopathic Pharmacopoeia* of the time from the tests for safety and efficacy required for other drugs. Thus, homeopathic remedies could be sold without first being studied and found safe and effective.

About 95 percent of homeopathic remedies are sold over the counter, which means that, by law, their use is limited to conditions that typically go away without any treatment and do not require diagnosis by a physician. However, the recent rise in the popularity of homeopathy has been accompanied by increasing numbers of unsubstantiated claims for homeopathic remedies against serious and chronic illnesses. Even homeopathic organizations have decried these claims, because they could keep people from getting appropriate help promptly for serious diseases in which time is crucial.

Consumer Reports magazine has joined other public protection groups in urging Congress to remove the exemptions from drug laws enjoyed by homeopathic remedies, so that homeopathic remedies, like others, must be shown to work and to be safe before they are marketed.

Some contemporary homeopaths suggest that Hahne-mann's "vital force" also might involve immune activity, but that has not yet been scientifically shown. Other proponents lean on the beliefs of Ayurvedic and Chinese healing traditions, suggesting that homeopathic remedies create an internal order that promotes good health. The existence of electromagnetic or subtle energy of the original substance's memory is not supported by scientific study.

Clinical homeopathic research addresses the question of whether human ailments respond to homeopathic preparations, regardless of any mechanism that may or may not lie behind homeopathic activity. One homeopathic study has merited publication in a peer-reviewed U.S. medical journal. That study concerned diarrhea in infants, and it was heavily criticized for biases that could have produced positive results by chance. More than one study concerning any particular health problem must produce the same results before a remedy is considered adequately tested. Scientifically acceptable proof of homeopathy's effectiveness awaits that further testing.

What It Can Do for You

Most scientists say that homeopathic remedies are essentially water and can act only as placebos, which heal indirectly through mental suggestion (see Chapter 19). However, homeopathic remedies offer the opportunity for self-care using nonaddicting products that are safe and have no side effects. If only through the power of the mind, they can be used to reduce the symptoms of self-limiting illnesses (problems such as aches and pains that will go away on their own in a week or so). Homeopathic remedies help many people get through these problems with fewer symptoms, and the treatments may shorten the length of these illnesses.

Many avid proponents swear by homeopathic remedies for allergies, colds and flu, and other minor but extremely annoying ailments. Homeopathic remedies have not been shown to have any impact on serious illness. In fact, using homeopathic remedies may delay diagnosis and standard treatment of serious illness when time is of the essence. Homeopathy's only danger

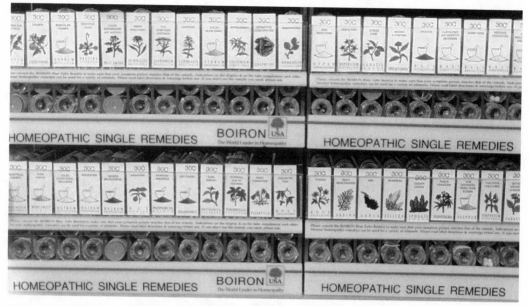

Figure 7 Dozens of tiny bottles fill the shelves of this pharmacy's homeopathic remedy section.

lies in postponing more targeted, conventional treatment for major diseases such as cancer that are best caught and treated as early as possible.

Where to Get It

+ Medical doctors (M.D.s) who practice homeopathic medicine may so advertise themselves in telephone book listings, typically under "family" or "general practice" physicians. Health-food stores and shops that carry homeopathic products (Figure 7) usually can provide names of homeopathic practitioners.

+ The National Center for Homeopathy in Alexandria, Virginia (703 548-7790), offers information as well as practitioner referrals.

+ Homeopathic books and tapes are available at Homeopathic Educational Services in Berkeley, California (800 359-9051).

+ The International Foundation for Homeopathy in Seattle, Washington (206 324-8230), provides referrals and educational programs.

5
Native American Healing

The first Americans were Eurasians who crossed the Bering Strait landbridge that linked Siberia with Alaska over 30,000 years ago. They worked their way south, eventually to settle the Americas. Some became the Native American tribes that developed the first communities and civilizations throughout North America.

Over thousands of years during which time these groups developed independently and often distantly from one another, they created distinct cultural and healing practices. Despite the differences, however, their common Eurasian origin provided a thread of commonality that remains to this day. Most of their practices and beliefs share important characteristics that link them not only with each other but also with the ancient healing systems that eventually became codified as Asian medicine. These features include the merging of medicine and religion, belief in an integral relationship between the person, the environment, and the cosmos, related assumptions about the role played by spiritual forces in health and disease, herbal remedies, purging rituals, and the involvement of shamans. **Shamans** are trained spiritual healers—often women—who served as the focus of ancient Asian as well as Native American medicine (See Chapter 53).

What It Is

Native American medicine is a system of healing used today by many as a primary source of medical care, and by others in combination with Western medicine. As in ancient Ayurvedic and Chinese medicine (see Chapters 2 and 3), Native American healing practices not only treat disease but are also employed to promote harmony among people in the community and between the physical environment and the spiritual world.

Native American healing has major mystical components. It does not differentiate between medicine, religion, spirituality, and magic. Physical illness typically is attributed to spiritual causes. Healing involves activities that will appease the spirits, rid the individual of impurities, and restore a healthful, spiritually pure state.

Shaman

A likely source for this word is the Mongolian adaptation of the Chinese term meaning "priest doctor." Used by northern Asian tribes, the word seems to have traveled from Siberia to describe Native American "medicine men."

With some variations across tribes, four predominant healing techniques are practiced by Native Americans: purifying and purging the body, the use of herbs, involvement of shamanic healers, and symbolic ritual. These four techniques are described below, with the understanding that modifications and embellishments occur from tribe to tribe.

Purification or **purging rituals**, similar to the practices found in other early healing systems and in other forms of folk medicine, remain important aspects of Native American healing. A traditional Native American purging ritual occurs in the sweat lodge. Here, heated rocks are doused with water, producing copious amounts of steam and heat that cause profuse sweating in those seated around the rocks. The sweating is thought to purge and purify the body. Southeastern tribes pursued an additional type of purging. They practiced the ancient Asian and Indian tradition of induced vomiting, with the help of an herbal tea preparation called the "Black Drink."

Native Americans also developed a rich knowledge of **herbal medicine**. The Creek Indians, for example, learned to drink willow tea to ease aching joint pain. It is now known that willow tea contains salicin, the natural form of acetylsalicylic acid, which is the active ingredient in aspirin. Particular herbal preparations vary from tribe to tribe.

A shaman might be employed when self-medication or therapy obtained from a trained herbalist proves insufficient to cure or slow an illness. Shamans, also called "medicine men" (although many are women), are trained healers thought to embody special powers in the spirit world. Prayers and ceremonies, important components of healing, usually are led by shamans. They are thought to be capable of invoking the healing powers of the spiritual forces, and also to appease those spirits who, angered by a patient, are believed to have caused the patient's illness.

Native American medicine includes a variety of **symbolic healing rituals**. One type exemplifies the communal nature of efforts to restore health. An example is the Dineh (Navaho) tribe's "sing," a community ceremony that can last from two days to more than a week. The chants are lengthy and complicated, requiring years to learn. Because learning the entire ritual of a chant is so arduous, most singers learn only a few in their lifetimes, and they tend to specialize in chants focused on a particular purpose. Some singers specialize in making the diagnosis, often using trances to determine the cause of a patient's illness. Once the cause is established, a singer who knows an appropriate chant is brought in to eliminate the disease. The preparation of herbal remedies and the creation of sand paintings, which are believed to promote healing, may accompany the chanting ceremony. The singer is responsible not only for the chant, but also for the preparation of herbs and paintings.

The Sioux (Lakota) have a set of seven healing ceremonies. One of the most dramatic is the Sun Dance, a four-day-long summer festival of prayer and ceremony. Sun dancers often are pierced: two cuts are made in the chest, and a wooden peg inserted through the cuts. This peg is tied to a tree which the dancer circles, connected to the tree by the stick threaded in his skin. The skin cuts are made by shamans, another example of the mingling of religion and medicine in Native American culture.

The Sioux also employ the Yuwipi, a spirit-calling ceremony often held for healing purposes. For the Yuwipi ceremony, the participant's hands are bound, and he is completely wrapped in a blanket tied around his body. The participant then implores the spirits, through prayer, to heal or perform some other task, such as locating missing persons.

What Practitioners Say It Does

The communal and spiritual essence of Native American healing finds many followers today among non-Native Americans in search of new religious experience. Native American healing is said to heal body and soul, appease ancestral spirits, evoke a sense of community concern for the sick individual, and help him or her as well as the entire group achieve a feeling of belonging.

Beliefs on Which It Is Based

Native American medicine rests on the core belief that all life is interconnected, and that everyone and everything has a corresponding presence in the spiritu-

Symbolic Healing Rituals

These include a colorful array of creative activities and objects such as sand painting (Navaho), chants, dances, drumming, medicine rattles; the medicine wheel or sacred hoop of the Lakota (Sioux), purifying the air by burning special herbs, and the Iroquois' use of masks to expel illness.

al world. Not only living things including plants and insects, but also inanimate objects such as rocks and wind, are believed to contain spirits. The web of life and the connectedness of body and spirit are fundamental to the related belief that the spirit world can influence the activities of the physical world, and thus promote health or cause illness. Shamans were employed primarily for their ability to access and influence the spiritual forces that govern the physical world.

Thoughts and ideas are believed to have the power to influence events. The Navaho and other tribes, therefore, do not speak of death and dying for fear of causing it to occur. In modern times, this inhibits planning and can create other difficulties when Native Americans are hospitalized with terminal illnesses.

Native American healing systems blur the line that Westerners draw between religion and medicine. For example, a common Native American practice, particularly for young men, was an exercise known as the **vision quest**. In the vision quest, a young man would travel away from home, out into the wilderness for several days of fasting and prayer. This ritual was assumed to encourage the spirits to provide the boy with a "vision" that would dictate the course of his life and his role in the life of the tribe. Many shamans and healers were called to their profession as the result of a vision quest.

Sweat-lodge ceremonies had a physical purpose: the purification of the body. Along with their accompanying prayer, however, they were meant also to encourage spiritual practice. A person needs to live in harmony not only with the elements of the physical world, but with the spiritual world.

Native American healing is characterized also by its communal nature. Many healing ceremonies are conducted in groups, and individual patients often are surrounded by chanting or praying family members when receiving treatment at home or in a hospital. This is in marked contrast to healing in many other systems, which presume a one-on-one relationship between caregiver and patient. It differs also from Western systems that encourage a high degree of confidentiality between doctor and patient.

Communal healing reflects the belief held by many Native American groups that an imbalance or disharmony in an individual is a threat to the harmony and well-being of the entire community. This view flows from the Native American emphasis on the interrelatedness of life and all of nature's creations, and on the overriding importance of the tribe as a whole.

Research Evidence to Date

Probably because of its fundamentally spiritual and magical nature, there has been almost no scientific study of Native American healing by Native American or other scientists. As in other ethnic healing systems, there are anecdotal reports of Native American healers curing serious disease. However, these reports have not been formally investigated.

What It Can Do for You

The effectiveness of Native American healing appears attributable primarily to psychological and mind-body influences. Native American ceremonies such as the sweat lodge and the vision quest may provoke insight and offer the chance for contemplation. These ceremonies are more spiritual than medical, and offer more in the way of introspection, insight, and revitalization than physical healing.

Some modern Americans, for example, whether or not of Native American heritage, have begun to study shamanism and engage in Native American spiritual practices. Typically they do this not to achieve medical healing, but to experience what the communal rituals offer, to achieve self-understanding and spiritual rejuvenation, and to obtain guidance for future courses of action.

These ceremonies may be combined with rituals and symbols from other sources. Some create a **kiva**, a round Pueblo ceremonial hut outdoors, in a special room, or in the basement of their homes. For a recent multicultural celebration of the spring equinox solstice, some friends of the author sat in their kiva, one facing west and the other east, on either side of a large, centrally placed quartz stone. They decided to bring rainbow light from deep within the womb of Mother Earth through the vortex of the quartz. Meditating, they soon saw ribbons of light and energy flooding the room. They shared their interpretations of this effect and concluded the three-hour ceremony shortly before midnight, feeling a sense of peace and connection with the universe.

Where to Get It

Many books about Native American rituals are available:

+ *Mother Earth Spirituality* (Harper & Row, San Francisco, 1990), by Ed McGaa (Eagle Man), describes several ceremonies at length, detailing their history and ritual. It offers instruction on how to construct a sweat lodge and make a peace pipe. Like other books about Native American healing, it focuses on spiritual healing.

+ John Neihardt's *Black Elk Speaks* (Pocket Books, New York, 1972) offers firsthand recollections of an Oglala Sioux healer.

+ Joseph Epes Brown's *The Sacred Pipe: Black Elk's Account of the Seven Rites of the Oglala Sioux*, (Penguin Books, Bergenfield, N.J., 1971) provides further insight into Native American religion and medicine through a study of Sioux rituals.

Some organizations, such as the Omega Institute in Rhinebeck, New York (914 266-4444), and the Foundation for Shamanic Studies in Mill Valley, California (415 380-8282) offer seminars in various aspects of Native American healing.

~6
Naturopathic Medicine

Naturopathic medicine is an approach to healing practiced by naturopathic doctors (N.D.s), who diagnose illness with the same techniques used by conventional physicians. They treat illness with natural methods, however, avoiding pharmaceutical drugs and other products of modern medicine. Naturopathy was organized in the late nineteenth century. By the early 1900s, there were more than twenty schools of naturopathic medicine in the United States, and naturopathic conventions in the 1920s often attracted more than 10,000 practitioners.

Most schools of naturopathy became defunct by the 1940s, however, when standards of quality were introduced, bringing increased scrutiny to medicine and the licensing of medical schools. Interest in naturopathy waned shortly thereafter. Today, however, naturopathy is among the many forms of alternative and complementary medicine enjoying a resurgence of interest.

What It Is

Naturopathic medicine, positioned as a low-cost, more gentle alternative to conventional care, combines modern knowledge of the body and disease with a variety of healing methods not used in mainstream medicine. The naturopathic approach to disease includes the many natural methods geared to strengthen the body's own healing ability. Treatment avoids drugs and surgery. Although naturopaths are not M.D.s, they do perform minor surgical procedures.

Unlike many alternative systems of care, naturopathic medicine does not have its own view of human physiology, function, and disease apart from that held by conventional medicine. Rather than relying on concepts such as the body types of Ayurvedic medicine or the vital life force concept of traditional Chinese medicine, naturopaths study conventional anatomy and other medical sciences. They use X rays, order laboratory tests, and apply physical examination techniques as do conventional physicians.

Naturopathy and conventional medicine differ, how-

Naturopathic Techniques and Areas of Care

- Therapeutic nutrition
- Homeopathy
- Plant substances
- Manipulation of muscles, bones, and spine
- Natural childbirth (not in hospital)
- Pre- and postnatal care
- Acupuncture and other techniques of traditional Chinese medicine
- Counseling
- Hypnotherapy
- Hydrotherapy
- Minor surgery

ever, in emphasis and treatment. Naturopathy is not associated with a unique healing technology. Rather, it uses a collection of natural treatment modalities such as botanical medicine, nutritional therapies, homeopathy, acupuncture, traditional Asian medicine, hydrotherapy, counseling, and physical medicine (manipulation of muscles and bones).

Homeopathy (see Chapter 4) is a system of medicine involving the use of very small amounts of a symptom-causing substance to treat the condition that produces similar symptoms. **Traditional Chinese medicine** (Chapter 3) applies techniques developed in ancient China to treat disease, and acupuncture (see Chapter 1) involves the insertion of needles in specific points on the body to cure or treat disease. For **hydrotherapy** or **spa therapy**, patients are sent to spas for periods of rest and rejuvenation. This is especially popular in Europe, and spa therapy is even covered by some European insurance programs.

The primary technique of physical medicine is a system of manipulating the bones and spine in a way that is similar to chiropractic and osteopathic manipulation. Physical forces such as electricity, heat, and sound also are applied to treat patients, as are various massage and exercise techniques.

Botanical medicine involves the use of whole plants and herbs as medicines, a practice with a long tradition in many cultures. Naturopathic physicians believe that botanical medicines are superior to synthetic drugs in some instances. They also claim that botanical medicines are safer, have fewer side effects, and are less costly.

Naturopaths use food as medicine, ensuring that each patient follows the optimum diet for his or her health and lifestyle. Healthful, nutritionally balanced diets are prescribed. Advocates point to increasing evidence about the role of nutrition in disease, and the extensive training in nutrition received by naturopathic doctors compared with conventional physicians.

Counseling or behavioral medicine is an important component of naturopathy, and practitioners emphasize the role played by mental and emotional health in disease. Naturopathic physicians are trained in counseling, biofeedback, stress reduction, and other means of helping improve mental and therefore overall health. Some naturopathic physicians obtain further training in one or more of these techniques and specialize in treating patients with these methods. Naturopathic doctors may also apply other alternative or unproven techniques, such as ozone therapy for patients with cancer or AIDS.

Acceptance requirements for naturopathic medical school are similar to those for mainstream medical schools. They include a college degree and the completion of courses in physics, biology, and chemistry. The first two years of school include conventional medical science such as anatomy, physiology, and pathology. The last two years are devoted to the specific techniques of naturopathic treatment discussed above, and to seeing patients, primarily in outpatient (nonhospital) environments, under the supervision of fully trained and experienced naturopathic practitioners.

Training, however, is substantially different for N.D.s and M.D.s. While conventional physicians undergo four years of training as do naturopathic physicians, conventional physicians must also serve a minimum of three years of residency after medical school before they may practice. The additional three years plus passing required tests allow them to practice only general or family medicine. The practice of a medical specialty such as cardiology, oncology, or pediatrics, requires several additional years of study.

Naturopathic physicians who pass certifying exams offered by the Council on Naturopathic Medical Education, in contrast, are licensed and may begin practice directly after their four-year program. There are no residency or additional training requirements.

What Practitioners Say It Does

Naturopaths view naturopathic medicine as an alternative to conventional primary care, claiming to treat the same range of illnesses and referring patients to other conventional specialists as necessary. Naturopaths do not provide emergency care and they do not perform major surgery. Some naturopathic physicians practice natural childbirth in the home or at a birthing center. However, naturopathic medicine claims to treat almost the entire range of illness, from self-limiting and minor

Migraine headaches: evening prim-
rose oil.

Chronic lower back pain: acupuncture.

Enlarged prostate: saw palmetto
herb.

Menopause symptoms: botanical
formula.

conditions to major life-threatening illnesses such as
AIDS and cancer.

Proponents stress that naturopathic therapy has fewer
side effects and lower costs than conventional medicine.
Some of these differences, however, may be due to the
fact that naturopaths refer complicated cases or patients
requiring major treatment to conventional practitioners.
For example, naturopaths are unable to handle problematic births, referring such cases to hospital-based obste-
tricians.

Beliefs on Which It Is Based

Naturopathy's overarching goal is to enlist the natural
healing power of the body to fight disease. Some naturopaths equate this healing power with the "vital force"
idea that underlies the traditional healing systems from
many ancient cultures. A related emphasis is placed on
uncovering and treating the cause of disease instead of
merely alleviating symptoms.

Other naturopathic principles include avoiding drugs
and surgery in favor of natural methods. Through
detailed examination of the patient's lifestyle and medical history, naturopathic physicians emphasize treating
the whole person and understanding his or her overall
lifestyle, environment, and the interactions that will
influence well-being.

Naturopathy also emphasizes preventive medicine.
Patients are taught to adopt healthful diets and lifestyles
in an effort to ward off the development of illness. To
this end, naturopathic doctors are seen as teachers who
educate patients about their own bodies and about the
best ways to maintain health. Naturopathy's beliefs and
methods stem from case-history observations, medical
records, practitioners' experience in treating patients,
clinical nutritional data, and therapies long popular in
Europe, Asia, and India.

Research Evidence to Date

Naturopathic medicine uses several specific techniques that vary in their effectiveness or ability to influence health. Some naturopathic approaches, such as
homeopathy, may be of little value. Others are documented and known to be effective. Examples include

the importance of diet in modifying the risk of severe illnesses such as heart disease and cancer, and the use of acupuncture to reduce pain and to assist withdrawal from addiction.

Researchers at the University of Minnesota Medical School examined naturopathic treatments and found some supporting scientific evidence in their favor, plus the need for definitive clinical trials.

Naturopathic medicine is an excellent example of how the nature of proof can differ between conventional and alternative physicians. Most techniques used by naturopathic physicians have long traditions, and practitioners cite these traditions as evidence of effectiveness. Conventional medicine requires validation of therapies with clinical trials.

What It Can Do for You

Because naturopathy uses many different techniques, it is necessary to examine them individually, just as conventional medical therapy would be evaluated. Most naturopathic remedies are considered harmless by conventional practitioners, but more study is needed before naturopathic therapies can be said to reverse disease.

Naturopathic treatments generally can be helpful against minor illnesses, but using naturopathic instead of conventional therapy for major illnesses or serious conditions is not wise.

Where to Get It

There are over 1,000 licensed naturopathic doctors (N.D.s) and two accredited naturopathic medical schools in the United States. These are the Bastyr College of Naturopathic Medicine in Seattle, which recently changed its name to Bastyr University, and the National College of Naturopathic Medicine in Portland, Oregon. Two additional schools, in Toronto, Canada, and Scottsdale, Arizona, are active candidates for accreditation but not yet accredited. The American Association of Naturopathic Physicians and the National Institutes of Health (NIH) Office of Alternative Medicine can provide information describing naturopathic training.

As this distribution of schools suggests, the Pacific Northwest is a stronghold of naturopathic medicine in

As of 1995, ten states and the District of Columbia licensed naturopathic physicians:

Alaska	New Hampshire
Arizona	Montana
Connecticut	Oregon
Florida	Utah
Hawaii	Washington

Florida and Utah, however, no longer license new N.D.s.

the United States. In fact, Oregon has more accredited naturopathic physicians than any other state. Accreditation is provided by the American Association of Naturopathic Physicians (AANP), naturopathy's national professional organization.

The AANP strongly recommends that patients verify their naturopathic physician's certification with the AANP. The AANP warns that some practitioners who advertise themselves as N.D.s obtained degrees in courses at unaccredited schools or through the mail, rather than at accredited institutions. Naturopaths are licensed in ten states in the United States (see box), but practice in at least twenty-eight additional states.

To find a naturopath in your area, contact the AANP by phone (206 323-7610) or by mail (P.O. Box 20386, Seattle, WA 98102). AANP also maintains a World Wide Web site (www.infinity.dorsai.org/naturopathic.physician), which contains a directory of naturopathic physicians by state, as well as other information about naturopathic medicine and naturopathic medical schools.

Approximately 100 insurance companies in the United States and Canada cover naturopathic care. A few insurance companies now offer subscribers a choice between naturopathic and conventional services. These programs use naturopaths as primary-care doctors who maintain responsibility for patients' overall care and refer patients to mainstream medical specialists as necessary.

Seattle's American Western Life, for example, offers a "Wellness Plan" that employs naturopathic physicians. Enrollees in the plan undergo mandatory checkups with naturopathic physicians, and have access to other alternative healers such as homeopaths and aromatherapists. The plan also offers access to a natural products pharmacy.

Similarly, Blue Cross of Washington and Alaska introduced "AlternaPath" on a pilot basis in 1994. It provides access to both mainstream and alternative practitioners. Subscriber demand and customer satisfaction have led Blue Cross to offer this program on a wider basis. The state of Washington requires health insurers to cover acupuncture, massage therapy, and other types of licensed natural health care.

PART TWO

DIETARY AND HERBAL REMEDIES

Alternative dietary approaches run the gamut from extremist nutritional "cancer cures," such as the grape diet, to healthful living approaches also encouraged by mainstream wellness proponents. Can food be used as medicine?

Hippocrates thought so. Let food be your medicine, counseled the famed fifth-century B.C. Greek physician. His dictum is followed today, not only by responsible nutrition experts seeking to change the way Americans eat, but also by exploiters and misguided souls who make outlandish claims for fad diets, massive doses of vitamins, and costly untested supplements.

In this section you will find evangelists—proponents of special diets who couple a faith in dietary efficacy with appeals to nature or the spirit. Advocates of macrobiotics believe that their limited fare and strictures against certain utensils lead not only to improved health but also to spiritual harmony with the world. Fasting, a practice used in a limited way across religions for millennia as a method to cleanse the soul, is thought by its advocates to cleanse and heal the body as well.

Indeed, there is a very real need for Americans to improve their diets, and often the advice of alternative diet proponents is consistent with sound nutritional evidence. Consensus agreement among nutritionists and physicians who specialize in nutrition science is edging toward the low-fat, high-fiber, plant- and carbohydrate-based diet that some proponents of dietary alternatives have advocated for years.

Phytomedicine, a legitimate branch of pharmaceutical study, is based on herbs and herbal derivatives and synthetics, and includes everything from pain relievers to chemotherapy. This practice merges ancient herbal tradition with modern scientific investigation. It also describes a coming together of the popular interest in "natural" healthy foods and the knowledge of modern science that supports many of those traditional beliefs.

The alternatives described in this section may contradict, complement, or stand outside the sphere of conventional nutrition. In some instances, various approaches contradict one another. For example, a macrobiotic diet has a vegetarian basis, but many advocates of vegetarianism find it nutritionally deficient.

Advocates of both vitamins and **orthomolecular medicine** (the use of extremely high doses of vitamins as therapy) agree that vitamin supplements enhance health, at least under some circumstances, but they disagree on the amounts necessary to accomplish the goal. As happens in other areas of alternative healing, many proponents of dietary cures take a grain of fact and use it to bake a loaf of unsupported conclusions.

Dietary recommendations are based on three facts. First, what we eat undeniably affects our health. Studies have found that diets rich in fiber, fruits, and vegetables can not only reduce obesity, but also lower the risk of heart disease and certain types of cancer. Vitamin substitutes for the foods themselves do not accomplish these same preventive goals. Conversely, diets high in calories and fat, particularly saturated fat, can lead to chronic diseases and morbidity. Second, the diets of many Americans do not resemble this low-fat, high-fiber ideal. Our affluence has led us to diets that contain too much fat, too little fiber, and excessive calories. All of this contributes to high rates of heart disease and record levels of obesity in the population.

Third, the nature of dietary advice evolves as addi-

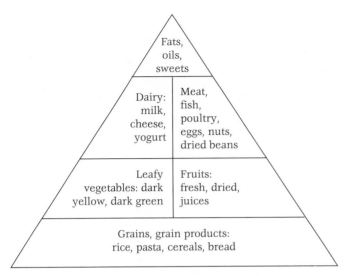

Figure 8 The USDA guidelines for daily healthful eating, as symbolized by this food pyramid, include 6 to 11 servings of grains; 2 to 5 servings each of vegetables and fruits; 2 to 3 servings of dairy products; 2 to 3 servings of meat, poultry, nuts, or eggs; and very small amounts of fats, oils, and sweets.

tional scientific information is uncovered. The food pyramid put out by the U. S. Department of Agriculture (USDA) reflects the latest consensus on balanced nutrition. Today's food pyramid (Figure 8) places more emphasis on fiber, grains, fruits, and vegetables and less on the protein, meat, and dairy products than was emphasized in earlier government guidelines. This increased focus on plant-based foods and carbohydrates is consistent with beliefs long propounded by vegetarians, who proclaim the benefits of a plant-based, low-fat diet. Changes in the government's dietary advice are made according to carefully controlled scientific studies.

Many alternative and fad diets are either not scientifically validated or are marketed despite having been found worthless or harmful. Diets that include only one food—grapefruit or beefsteak, for example— are antithetical to two basic principles of good nutrition: moderation and variety.

The claims made in support of dietary therapies vary widely. Some diets are said to be more in harmony with nature, or to better align one's physical and spiritual self than others, and therefore to yield spiritual benefits. Herbs and other dietary supplements often are marketed on the incorrect claim that natural products are safer and produce fewer side effects than prescription or over-the-counter (OTC) drugs. Fasting is promoted as a "natural" method for the elimination of toxins, but evidence for the existence and specifics of these toxins is nowhere in sight.

Other bases for alternative diets include ancient tradition, both medical and cultural. It has long been known that certain foods can prevent disease. For example, eating fruits and vegetables prevents scurvy. Modern scientists discovered that scurvy is caused by a vitamin C deficiency, which eating fruits and vegetables can prevent. Advocates of high-dose vitamin regimens take the fact that vitamin deficiencies cause disease, and extrapolate to the conclusion that megadoses of vitamins prevent or cure disease.

Nobel Laureate Linus Pauling, Ph.D., for example, famous for his work as a chemist and worker for world peace, in his later career advocated massive doses of vitamin C to prevent cancer. This view, still espoused by many of his supporters, is not backed by any evidence according to mainstream scientists.

Ancient healing systems such as India's Ayurvedic medicine and traditional Chinese medicine (Chapters 2 and 3) include dietary remedies. Plants and herbs were the first medicines in every culture. Modern alternative remedies, such as the diet- and coffee-enema-based metabolic therapies as well as other unproven cancer regimens, also include special diets.

Healthful eating keeps us in good shape and prevents many illnesses. However, aside from diseases of nutritional deficiency, there are no proven dietary cures for serious illnesses.

Herbal and dietary supplements that claim to enhance strength or prolong youth or improve memory are permitted to appear on your local grocery and health-store shelves bearing no information about their safety and effectiveness. In contrast, pharmaceutical and medical device companies must go through strict and lengthy processes to prove that their products are safe and that they work before they are permitted to bring them to market.

The inescapable fact is that how we eat influences how we feel and how well our bodies are equipped to ward off major disease. As important as diet turns out to be, the companion fact is that food does not cure serious illness. Don't be fooled into substituting a special diet for real medical treatment when it is needed to save your life.

7

Regulatory Issues: Who's Minding the Store?

When you go to the drug store for aspirin today, you can be reasonably sure that what you're buying is safe and that it contains no more or less than what the package says it contains. It was not always that way with pharmaceuticals, and it still is not that way with health-food products and dietary supplements sold in health-food stores, supermarkets, and pharmacies.

Despite continuing concern on the part of Food and Drug Administration (FDA) officials and others who work in the public interest, there are still no across-the-board standards or federal laws governing the quality of food supplements, herbs, and other products marketed with claims for improving health benefits. *Caveat emptor*—let the buyer beware—is the only rule governing the purchase of many products used as health foods or dietary supplements. What you think you are buying is not necessarily what you get.

Laws and regulations regarding the manufacture, promotion, and sale of foods and drugs were needed initially in the early years of this century, when profiteering and fraud were rampant. Food was often contaminated, adulterated with harmful chemicals, and packaged under unsanitary conditions. Worthless "medicines" were sold as cure-alls by pseudodoctors and traveling "snake oil" salesmen. They were also promoted in newspaper ads and sold through the mail.

Labeling was deceptive and rarely indicated what the products actually contained. Outrageous claims of curative powers for everything from colds to cancer dominated the packaged medicine field. Practices in both the food and drug industries were dangerous as well as deplorable.

The federal government finally took action resulting in the innovative and much-needed Food and Drugs Act of 1906. Although the act did away with misbranding and adulteration, it left intact a serious problem: the safety and effectiveness of drugs. Were they safe or harmful? Did they live up to their claims or accomplish nothing? Did they produce side effects, causing the risk to outweigh any benefit? Drug manufacturers were not obliged to report information about safety and efficacy, nor were they required even to test their products to see if they were safe and effective. All claims were made with impunity.

It took two disasters, twenty-five years apart, before the federal government properly addressed safety concerns. The first occurred in 1937, when a Tennessee company developed a liquid form of a sulfa medicine. Called Elixir Sulfanilamide, the product was developed for those who preferred to drink their medicine. It was marketed without prior testing for toxicity. The liquid base, diethylene glycol, turned out to be poisonous, causing kidney failure and death in 105 people.

An angry public demanded better protection, and a year later the Federal Food, Drug, and Cosmetic Act was passed. This act banned false and misleading statements on labels for food, drugs, and medical devices. It also required proof of safety for drugs entering interstate commerce. However, drugs already on the market and covered by the 1906 act were grandfathered, and therefore proof of safety was not required from them. The act helped, but much stronger and broader regulation was still needed.

The thalidomide tragedy precipitated the additional needed regulation. This drug was manufactured by a German company for use as a sedative in 1953. Almost 40 percent of the women who took thalidomide during pregnancy, mainly in European countries where the drug was first introduced, delivered seriously malformed babies who typically lacked limbs. Pictures of the infants without arms were shown almost daily in the news media. People were aghast that so many innocent women and children paid such a high price for industry's failure to properly test the products it brought to market. (A similar tragedy occurred in the early 1970s, when the long-term effects of DES, a synthetic female hormone used to prevent likely spontaneous abortion and premature labor, were found to increase vaginal and cervical cancer in daughters born to women who took DES during pregnancy.)

The link between these terrible tragedies and the drugs that caused them became evident in the early 1960s, just as the American pharmaceutical industry was under Congressional review in an investigation headed by Senator Estes Kefauver of Tennessee. The result was passage of the Drug Amendments of 1962, also called the Kefauver-Harris Amendments.

The new requirements dealt squarely with the problem that the thalidomide and Elixir Sulfanilamide disasters had so clearly demonstrated. Before any new drug, or any drug marketed after 1938 could be sold in the United States, it had to be proven both safe and effective. The amendments also gave the FDA the power to police the industry and enforce these regulations. The National Academy of Sciences was brought in to assist with this gargantuan task. One of the seventeen panels it developed was responsible for over-the-counter (OTC) drugs, a category that includes most dietary supplements and herbal products.

Because it was impossible to study and evaluate the hundreds of thousands of existing OTC drugs in short order, the FDA attempted to regulate them immediately by permitting their sale only if the label did not claim to prevent or treat disease. Eventually, some drugs were studied and reclassified when found to be unsafe or when their effectiveness was documented or disproved.

Most dietary supplements and herbs, however, continued to be sold, minus the now-illegal promises, as

---

The Supplement Shambles

Top experts in herbal medicine and dietary supplements decry the lack of public protection. The 1994 regulations take good care of the multibillion-dollar supplements industry, but they leave the consumer in the lurch. Here's what the November 1995 issue of *Consumer Reports* said about what the new law allows:

· Products can be sold with no testing for efficacy or effectiveness.

· Supplement manufacturers do not have to prove the safety of their products already on the market. Now the burden is on the FDA to show, *after* people die or experience adverse effects, that the product is *not* safe.

· There are no standards that manufacturers must follow. Even quality control standards will not be introduced for at least two years.

· Although products may not explicitly claim to cure or prevent a disease, other, unproven claims can still adorn the package.

· Labels need not have much evidence behind them, and that evidence, called "substantiation," need not be revealed unless regulators challenge label claims.

· Packaging or marketing claims do not require FDA approval.

The Alternative Medicine Handbook

foods or nutritional supplements. Innuendos (rather than promises) of far-reaching benefits persist on many product labels. Such implicit claims are beyond reach of the law, however, because they are indirect rather than explicit. Claims are couched, for example, in comments from satisfied users who describe how the product cured their illness or produced other benefits.

Although the public needs the protection provided by accurate labeling, proof of safety, and evidence of benefit, the food supplement industry effectively prevented legislation from passage in the U.S. Congress in 1994. It accomplished this with a successful multimillion-dollar campaign urging Americans to "Write to Congress today, or kiss your supplements good-bye!" This false message resulted in passage of the Dietary Supplement and Health Education Act of 1994, which created a protected new category for the estimated 20,000 vitamins, herbs, minerals, and anything else that had been sold as a supplement before October 1994.

Despite very real dangers, the FDA is allowed to halt production of a product not when the manufacturer fails to show that it is safe and effective, but only after the FDA itself proves the product to be dangerous to people's health.

The FDA is one of three government agencies with the authority to regulate the marketing of products we ingest. The U.S. Postal Service may police products marketed through the mail, and in recent times has challenged the sale of products promising cancer cures. The Federal Trade Commission has the authority to regulate the advertising of food, cosmetics, nonprescription products, and health-related services that are marketed across state lines.

Individual states also have some regulatory authority, through their licensing of health professionals and enactment of consumer protection laws. State licensing boards keep an eye out for harmful medical and dental practices, but they usually take years to investigate and terminate inappropriate activity. Some states have new and amended regulations governing alternative and complementary therapies, allowing physicians to use unproven treatments if the patient wants them and the physician feels they may help.

Today, clever promotional techniques and unproven product claims abound. The public is confronted with confusing information accompanied by innuendos of benefit unsupported by reliable data.

Some pharmacists join many Americans in feeling confused and coming to incorrect conclusions about OTC products. We consumers tend to believe that products sold over the counter are protected by governmental safeguards and therefore are safe for us to use. That is not the case, and OTC herbs and supplements remain very much in need of regulatory reform to protect not the industry but the public.

With current federal laws, consumer protection and enforcement agencies cannot provide adequate public protection against contaminated products, false indications of miracle results, and other dangers inherent in numerous dietary and herbal supplements. Store shelves contain many harmful and worthless products sold under false pretenses. They also offer a wide range of genuinely useful and safe products that can quicken relief of temporary ailments and improve quality of life. The challenge is to figure out which products are which. Until we are protected by better governmental regulations, the consumer is obliged to read labels carefully, check with accredited nutritionists and dietitians, and use good common sense.

8
Dietary Supplements

Thirteen vitamins and eighteen minerals are essential to life and health; a chart describing all the vitamins and most minerals concludes this chapter. Despite the fact that only milligrams—tiny, minute amounts—of each vitamin are needed, vitamins are essential to all of the body's biochemical processes. They are required to convert food into energy and to help the body manufacture hormones, blood cells, and nervous system chemicals.

Except for three—D, B_5, and B_7, which come in part from other sources—vitamins are obtained entirely from food. Pantothenic acid (B_5) and vitamin D can be produced by the absorption of sunlight through the skin. Ten minutes of exposure to the bright midday sun produces at least half of what adults require each day. The remainder must be consumed from fatty fish, such as salmon and tuna, and from dairy products. Some of the needed biotin (B_7) and pantothenic acid is produced by normal intestinal bacteria; remaining amounts are easily obtained from food.

Minerals are closely related to vitamins. They originate in soil and water, and are found in all plants and animals. The **major** (or **macro**) **minerals**, those needed in relatively large quantities by the body, include calcium, phosphorus, and magnesium. **Trace** (or **micro**) **minerals** are needed in very small amounts. Iron, fluoride, selenium, and zinc are among the eighteen essential trace minerals. Vitamins and minerals work together, influencing how well the body absorbs both.

Vitamins and minerals have been studied for decades, and a great deal is known about the sources and roles of each, as well as about what happens when the body takes in too much or too little of a particular substance. This information is given in the chart at the end of the chapter.

Scientists continue research in this area, working to expand knowledge about the effects of vitamins and minerals on health and physiological functioning, or learning that a bit more or less of a nutrient can produce better results than had been assumed. This is why the Recommended Dietary (or Daily) Allowances (RDAs) are reviewed regularly by the Food and Nutrition Board of

Basic Facts about Vitamins

· Vitamins come from animal or plant foods and are essential to human life and health.

· Four of the thirteen vitamins (A, D, E, K) are fat-soluble. Excess amounts are absorbed by body fat and stored for later use in case the body runs short of them in the future. Therefore, taking large amounts of A, D, E, and K as supplements can cause excessive accumulations of these vitamins that can be toxic.

· The remaining nine vitamins (C and the eight B vitamins) are water-soluble. This means they dissolve in body fluids, and the body eliminates excess amounts of them in the urine.

· All vitamins are designated by both letter and scientific names. By convention, some are called primarily by their letters (for example, C and D), while others are known more frequently by their scientific names (such as pantothenic acid (B_5) and biotin (B_7).

Vitamins and minerals interact in complex ways. Here are a few examples:

• The absorption of iron is enhanced by vitamin C, but too much vitamin C interferes with the body's ability to absorb copper, which is essential to body chemistry.

• Excessive amounts of B1 can cause deficiencies in B2 and B6.

• Too much phosphorus hurts calcium absorption.

• Absorption of copper and iron is inhibited by long-term use of zinc supplements.

Be wary of under- or overdosing. Instead, eat a balanced diet; follow RDA (Recommended Dietary Allowance) guidelines.

Deception?

Nutrition experts say we consumers have been taken in by the food supplement industry, buying vitamins and minerals in excess of need or when high doses may be harmful.

the National Research Council of the National Academy of Sciences. The reviews produce updated food guides, most recently a modified food pyramid shown in Figure 8 (page 57). The pyramid indicates the amount of each type of food required to meet the recommended RDAs.

What It Is

Vitamin supplements are purchased by up to 80 percent of U.S. households, and spending for vitamin capsules averages approximately $66 each year per household. Despite such widespread use, serious debate continues about the value of vitamin pills and other dietary supplements for the general public.

Scientific studies indicate that the necessary nutrients are provided by the average balanced diet, and that only certain groups of people require supplements: pregnant women, young children, alcoholics, those with diseases that inhibit absorption of nutrients, postmenopausal women trying to prevent osteoporosis, and people whose diets do not provide the required nutrients.

Recent studies, however, show that less than one-third of adults eat 5 servings of fruit and vegetables a day, and many older people consume fewer calories than required to meet daily nutrient requirements.

In addition to general vitamin supplements sold to compensate for less-than-ideal eating habits, supplements are promoted as insurance against inadequate intake of essential nutrients, including proteins. Other supplements focus on people's special needs, such as improved athletic performance, desire for thicker hair, or hopes of losing weight.

To the dismay of the related National Institutes of Health (NIH) programs and patient advocacy groups (such as those for the elderly and those that seek to protect patients with specific diseases such as Alzheimer's disease, mental illness, or cancer), many products claim to reduce or cure problems such as depression, sleep disorders, diminishing memory, cancer, indigestion, and arthritis. Still others promise to achieve antiaging effects, rejuvenation, and the elimination of toxins from the body. Literally hundreds of dietary supplements, nutritional aids, and similar products are widely promoted and generally available to the public. Their promises are rarely substantiated in fact.

A dietary supplement act passed in 1994 removed dietary and nutritional supplements from Food and Drug Administration (FDA) review. Therefore, supplements are not regulated. They are not evaluated for safety or purity, nor are they studied to see whether they live up to promoters' claims (see Chapter 7). Many ads for special supplements do not list ingredients, so the buyer does not know what is contained in the capsules that promise results such as improved eyesight or greater stamina.

The extensive, alternative use of nutritional supplements contrasts ironically with the simultaneous, popular emphasis on "natural" foods and the benefits of vegetables and wholesome diets.

What Practitioners Say It Does

Proponents of dietary supplements believe that people in general can benefit from nutritional aids. They recommend daily doses of vitamins and other nutrients to sustain health, prevent disease, and even cure illness.

Megavitamin and Orthomolecular Therapy

Scientific data on problems associated with deficiencies or overdoses of nutrients are well established, and vitamin and mineral supplements are used appropriately to compensate for vitamin *deficiencies*. But some alternative practitioners believe that huge dosages of vitamins, sometimes hundreds of supplement pills a day, can *cure disease*. These individuals practice **megavitamin** or **orthomolecular therapy** (the latter adds minerals and other nutrients), unproven methods considered dangerous by mainstream scientists.

In the 1950s, two psychiatrists theorized that a biochemical abnormality causes schizophrenia (it is now known that genetic defects are responsible). They administered large doses of niacin and C, creating "mega (large dose) vitamin therapy." In 1968 the Nobel-prize-winning scientist Linus Pauling coined the term "orthomolecular" to describe the treatment of disease with large quantities of nutrients. His claims that massive doses of vitamin C could cure cancer were disproved in three clinical trials conducted at the Mayo Clinic.

Megavitamin therapists treat patients who have cancer, diabetes, schizophrenia, AIDS, pneumonia, flu, learning disabilities, depression, aging, autism, skin problems, hyperactivity, mental retardation, arthritis, and other diseases. The American Psychiatric Association and the NIH issued statements about megavitamin or orthomolecular therapies for psychiatric diseases, calling them and their unsubstantiated promotion ineffective, harmful, and deplorable.

Although megadoses of some vitamins can cause serious toxic effects (see the chart at the end of this chapter), an even more serious problem is that patients with major, treatable diseases may turn to megavitamin therapy instead of mainstream care. This was shown in a recent television documentary, in which a young woman with treatable breast cancer rejected surgery to remove the tumor in favor of megadoses of vitamins.

Scientific research has found no benefit to orthomolecular therapy for any disease.

Recommended Dietary Allowances (RDAs) for Vitamin and Mineral Intake

· RDAs are set by the FDA, based on studies by the National Academy of Sciences.

· Although some people assume these to be minimum standards, they are actually safe maximum standards.

· RDAs are generally well above the level at which deficiency occurs, and below the level at which harm occurs.

· RDAs usually are given in milligrams, but some are still reported in the older International Units (IU).

· Some essential nutrients are not yet evaluated for RDAs, but are assigned Estimated Minimum Daily Requirements (EMDR).

Why Does Coffee Smell So Good?

Perhaps we're drawn to drink it because it contains antioxidants— comparable to those found in fruits and vegetables!

In addition, extra products are suggested to achieve results that most would find desirable, such as increased vitality and enhanced well-being.

Beliefs on Which It Is Based

It is the opinion of megadose advocates that most people require vitamins and minerals in much greater amounts than they receive through their diets, and in dosages often far greater than their RDAs. They believe that, when it comes to vitamins and minerals, if some is good, more must be better. Typically these beliefs are not substantiated; often they are voiced by purveyors of food supplements who also promote a myriad of over-the-counter remedies for a wide range of ailments and deficiencies.

Research Evidence to Date

Research has shown that people who are nutritionally deficient benefit from supplements. It is well established that a daily vitamin can compensate for iron deficiency in menstruating women and for poor diets in the frail elderly. Pregnant women require at least 50 percent higher levels of vitamins than usual, plus extra vitamin D and folic acid. Professional advice should be sought.

As of the late 1990s, antioxidants—vitamins C, E, and beta carotene (which the body converts to vitamin A)— starred as some of the most popular supplements. They were thought to provide protection against heart disease and cancer, and were widely available at health-food stores and pharmacies. The antioxidant story is a good example of why large and thorough studies are necessary before we really know if something works.

Antioxidant supplements became popular because studies showed less cancer and heart disease among people who ate more fruit and beta carotene-rich vegetables (dark leafy green, yellow, and orange vegetables) than among people who consumed fewer vegetables and fruits. That is still accurate, but antioxidant supplements turned out to be no substitute for the foods themselves. Three major studies, involving a total of 74,000 men and women, showed definitively that beta carotene supplements do not lower the risk of cancer or heart disease.

Among smokers in the studies, in fact, the beta carotene supplements increased the incidence of serious diseases. Supplements do not produce the same beneficial results seen with vegetables and fruits, probably because of currently unknown interactions with other helpful ingredients. No shortcuts here.

What It Can Do for You

A nutritionally healthy diet is essential to overall good health. Because the diets of many Americans are too inconsistent and too full of junk food to satisfy the body's nutritional needs, and because some people have special needs, supplements are sometimes required.

For example, despite the wide availability of folate, or folic acid, in poultry, green vegetables, citrus fruit, and other common foods (one fresh vegetable or fruit a day prevents folic acid deficiency), the diets of some pregnant women do not contain the 400 mcg (micrograms) of folic acid needed daily by pregnant women or the 200 mcg typically recommended for others. (A microgram is one millionth of a gram.) Folate is also associated with reduced risk of fatal coronary artery disease. Adding small amounts in the form of supplements provides the missing amount of folic acid needed to reduce the incidence of defective pregnancies and of heart disease, according to scientific studies.

Using supplements ensures meeting the RDA requirements, especially for those who are chronically ill, alcoholic, or who suffer from other conditions that impair their ability to eat or absorb necessary nutrients. If you have or may have a serious illness or a special condition such as pregnancy, seek professional attention. Do not attempt to treat yourself with megadoses of vitamins or minerals as recommended in popular "nutritional therapy" books.

There are important distinctions between dietary supplements in the form of the vitamin pill that many take each morning and products aimed at treating illness. A daily vitamin tablet is unnecessary if you eat a healthful, balanced diet, but it is good insurance against inadequate consumption of necessary nutrients in your food. A general daily supplement will help those whose diets do not provide the necessary nutrients or who have special needs, such as calcium to protect against osteoporosis.

Megadoses of certain nutrients, especially fat-soluble supplements such as beta carotene taken to prevent ill-

Vitamins, Minerals, and Colds

People seem to believe that **vitamin C** cures colds. But at least sixteen double-blind studies found no benefit. A classic study conducted by the University of Toronto divided 3,500 people into eight groups. Two groups each received 250, 1,000, or 2,000 mg of vitamin C daily; the final two groups got a placebo. Results: vitamin C did not prevent colds, but 250 mg, the amount in two glasses of orange juice, slightly decreased symptom severity for some; more than 250 mg produced no extra benefit. Bottom line: if only for minor or placebo effect, drink a few glasses of OJ or take 250 mg of C a day for your cold.

According to recent Cleveland Clinic research, **zinc** lozenges, bought over the counter and taken within 24 hours after the start of a cold, reduced symptoms and made the cold go away in 4.4 instead of 7.6 days. Good news!

ness, are quite another matter. They can be toxic, and they do not substitute for the nutrient protection obtainable directly from vegetables, fruits, garlic, fish, oat bran, soy products, and other foods associated with lower incidences of disease and longer life spans.

Nevertheless, many people, especially women, supplement their diets with extra calcium, vitamin E (because preliminary data suggest it may help prevent major diseases), and reasonable amounts of vitamin C. This appears to be a safe solution, avoiding overdoses and providing vitamin "insurance."

As for the ever-growing number of encapsulated promises—such as bee products to increase energy, chromium picolinate to decrease weight and increase muscle mass, "wellness" capsules with unnamed ingredient blends, and potency pills—their proponents' claims are not substantiated. These bottled promises, despite the fact that they do not work, have created a multibillion-dollar business out of the supplement industry.

Where to Get It

Newsletters produced by many major medical centers and respected organizations provide detailed, objective information about dietary supplements. These include:

+ *Harvard Health Letter,* P.O. Box 420300, Palm Coast, FL 32142 (800 829-9045)
+ *Mayo Clinic Health Letter,* P.O. Box 53889, Boulder, CO 80322 (800 333-9037)
+ *Tufts University Diet and Nutrition Letter,* P.O. Box 57857, Boulder, CO 80322 (800 274-7581)
+ *Environmental Nutrition,* P.O. Box 420451, Palm Coast, FL 32142-0451 (800 829-5384)
+ *UC Berkeley Wellness Letter,* P.O. Box 420148, Palm Coast FL 32142 (904 445-6414)
+ *Consumer Reports Health Letter,* P.O. Box 52148, Boulder, CO 80322

Major books on nutrition include:

+ *The Wellness Encyclopedia of Food and Nutrition,* edited by Sheldon Margen and the Editors of the University of California at Berkeley Wellness Letter (New York, Rebus, 1992).
+ *Total Nutrition: The Only Guide You'll Ever Need—From the Mount Sinai School of Medicine,* by Victor Herbert (New York, St. Martin's Press, 1994).

Osteoarthritis Remedy?

The combination of dietary supplements glucosamine and chrondroitin is said to reduce joint pain and produce greater joint flexibility. Anecdotal reports await substantiation by scientific studies.

Basic Vitamin and Mineral Information

VITAMINS

FAT-SOLUBLE

Fat-soluble vitamins can be stored by the body for later use, so they need not be consumed every day.

A

(retinoic acid, retinol, beta carotene)

RDA for Women: 4,000 IU or 2.4 mg (milligrams) beta carotene.
RDA for Men: 5,000 IU or 3 mg beta carotene.
Purpose: Maintains vision, bones, hair, teeth, glands, skin, reproduction; helps wound healing.
Source: Leafy green and yellow and orange vegetables; fruit; dairy products; organ meats.
Signs of Deficiency: Poor growth in children, poor resistance to infection, night blindness, dry skin.
Signs of Overdose: Joint and bone pain, birth defects, blurred vision, cracked skin, hair loss.
Supplement Needed? No. The body stores vitamin A for lengthy time; excess can cause problems.
History: First vitamin discovered.

D

(cholecalciferol, ergocalciferol)

RDA for Adults: 200 IU or 5 mcg (micrograms).
RDA for Children, Adolescents, Pregnant Women: 400 IU (10 mcg).
Purpose: Helps body absorb calcium and phosphorus; builds teeth and bones; helps muscle and nerve function; may keep osteoarthritis in check.
Source: Sunlight, fortified dairy products, organ meats, tuna, fish oil, egg yolks.
Signs of Deficiency: Rickets in children, soft bones, osteoporosis.
Signs of Overdose: Calcium deposits in heart, kidneys, blood vessels; hypertension.
Supplement Needed? No. Excess is stored and can be toxic.

E

(tocopherol compounds; an antioxidant)

RDA for Adults: 400 IU.
Purpose: Helps form muscles and red blood cells; ensures function of immune and endocrine systems and sex glands; deters hardening of arteries; lowers risk of heart attacks and cataracts.
Source: Green, leafy vegetables; whole grains, vegetable oils, seafood, eggs, nuts.
Signs of Deficiency: Rare: fluid retention, hemolytic anemia.
Signs of Overdose: Rare: reduced sexual function.
Supplement Needed? If diet does not provide. Excess does no harm except in extreme amounts (above 1,080 IU).

K

(menadione, phytonadione)

RDA for Women: 65 micrograms.
RDA for Men: 80 micrograms.
Purpose: Assists blood clotting, bone metabolism, kidney function.
Source: Half of needed amount made by intestinal bacteria; get rest from diet: green leafy vegetables, whole grains, potatoes, liver.
Signs of Deficiency: Bleeding, liver damage.

        Signs of Overdose: Yellow skin (jaundice in infants).

    Supplement Needed? Only by pregnant women and some babies. More than 500 micrograms can be toxic and must be prescribed by physician.

Excess amounts of water-soluble vitamins are typically excreted by the body in the urine. Therefore, the following vitamins should be consumed often if not daily.

B_1
(thiamine)

    RDA for Women: 1.1 mg (milligram).

    RDA for Men: 1.5 mg.

    Purpose: Promotes metabolism and digestion; helps nervous system function.

    Source: Whole grains and cereals, seafood, pork, potatoes, organ meats.

    Signs of Deficiency: Nausea, depression, anxiety, muscle cramps, irregular heart beats. Extreme: beriberi.

    Signs of Overdose: Deficiency of other B vitamins.

    Supplement Needed? If diet does not provide RDA, use multivitamin instead of B_1 supplement.

B_2
(riboflavin)

    RDA for Women: 1.3 mg (milligram).

    RDA for Pregnant Women: 1.6 mg.

    RDA for Men: 1.7 mg.

    Purpose: Helps release energy to cells; helps build red blood cells; needed for proper function of nerves, eyes, and adrenal glands.

    Source: Leafy green vegetables, fish, poultry, liver, organ meats.

    Signs of Deficiency: Mouth and nose sores, visual problems, difficulty swallowing.

    Signs of Overdose: Interferes with B_1 and B_6.

    Supplement Needed? Diet usually provides enough; B_2 supplements give too much, so fix diet instead.

NIACIN
(B_3)

    RDA for Women: 15 mg (milligram).

    RDA for Pregnant Women: 17 mg.

    RDA for Men: 19 mg.

    Purpose: Converts food to energy; synthesizes hormones, steroids, and fatty acids; supports gastrointestinal tract.

    Source: Seafood, poultry, seeds, nuts, fortified whole grains, potatoes.

    Signs of Deficiency: Diarrhea, mouth sores. Extreme deficiency (diarrhea, mental illness of pellagra) has been virtually eliminated in U.S. since fortification of breads and cereals with niacin.

    Signs of Overdose: Nausea, liver damage.

    Supplement Needed? Flour and other foods are niacin-enriched. Deficiency is most likely only in pregnant or lactating women, alcoholics, or patients with hyperthyroidism.

PANTO-
THENIC
ACID
(B5)

Estimated Minimum Daily Requirement (EMDR): 4 to 7 milligrams.
Purpose: Converts food to energy, builds red blood cells; makes adrenal hormones and chemicals that regulate nerve function.
Source: Made by intestinal bacteria; found in almost all plant and animal foods.
Signs of Deficiency: Unknown.
Signs of Overdose: Increases need for B_1, diarrhea, water retention.
Supplement Needed? No. Deficiency occurs only with extreme starvation.

B_6
(pyrodoxine)

RDA for Women: 1.6 mg (milligram).
RDA for Pregnant Women: 2.2 mg.
RDA for Men: 2 mg.
Purpose: Needed for protein and carbohydrate metabolism; forms red blood cells; promotes nerve function; supports immune function.
Source: Meat, fish, poultry, grains, spinach, bananas, prunes, watermelon, sweet potatoes, brown rice.
Signs of Deficiency: Depression, confusion, inflamed mouth membranes, scaly skin, convulsions in infants.
Signs of Overdose: Sensory nerve destruction: loss of feeling in legs, fingers, etc.
Supplement Needed? Too much or too little is dangerous; balanced diets provide right amount; deficiency occurs in those with malabsorption disorders.

BIOTIN
(B7,H)

Estimated Minimum Daily Requirement (EMDR): 30–100 mcg (micrograms).
Purpose: Metabolizes fatty acids and glucose; essential for many body processes.
Source: Found in almost all plant and animal foods.
Signs of Deficiency: Skin rash, hair loss, vomiting, inflamed tongue. Rare even in infancy, although breast milk contains little biotin.
Signs of Overdose: Deficiency of B_1 and B_6 .
Supplement Needed? No. Deficiency possible but rare in newborns; possible in long-term users of antibiotics.

FOLATE,
FOLIC
ACID
(B9)

RDA for Women and Men: 400 mcg (micrograms).
Purpose: Needed to make DNA, RNA, and blood cells; prevents neural tube defects; helps prevent deaths from coronary artery disease, may reduce risk of cancer.
Source: Dark leafy green vegetables, citrus fruit, poultry, liver. One fresh fruit or vegetable a day keeps deficiency away.
Signs of Deficiency: Anemia, weight loss. Deficiency seen in alcoholics, some pregnant women, the impoverished.
Signs of Overdose: Convulsions in epileptics, damages zinc absorption.
Supplement Needed? Yes, if you get less than 400 mcg from your diet. By 1998 the government will require increased folate supplementation in grain-based foods, cereals, and dietary supplements to reduce incidence of neural tube defects during fetal development.

B₁₂
(cobalamin)

RDA for Adults: 2 mcg (micrograms).
RDA for Pregnant Women: 2.2 mcg.
Purpose: Helps make red blood cells; builds genetic material needed by all cells; converts food to energy.
Source: All animal products: eggs, meat, poultry, seafood, low-fat dairy products; not in plants.
Signs of Deficiency: Weakness, sore tongue, tingling in arms and legs. Uncommon; usually limited to alcoholics, strict vegetarians, pregnant or nursing women, who should take supplements. Pernicious anemia results from severe deficiency.
Signs of Overdose: Considered nontoxic.
Supplement Needed? Yes for pregnant or nursing women. Deficiency uncommon; strict vegetarians and alcoholics may need supplements.

C
(ascorbic acid)

RDA for Adults: 200–400 mg (milligrams).
Purpose: Helps bones and teeth grow; binds cells together; helps resist infection; helps heal cuts and wounds; needed for blood clotting.
Source: Citrus and other fruits, sweet potatoes, cabbage, broccoli, peppers.
Signs of Deficiency: Bleeding gums, loose teeth, easy bruising, slow healing. Extreme cases: scurvy.
Signs of Overdose: Excess vitamin C is excreted in the urine. Side effects are uncommon: nausea, diarrhea, kidney stone formation.
Supplement Needed? If diet does not provide adequate amount. Because vitamin C is water-soluble, excess is excreted. May reduce symptoms but not length of colds

MINERALS

CALCIUM   *RDA for Adults:* 800–1000 mg (milligrams); 1,500 mg after age 65.
    RDA for Children: 800 mg.
        Purpose: Growth and maintenance of bones and teeth; enables heart and other muscle contraction.
        Source: Milk, canned salmon with bones, oysters, broccoli, tofu.
  Signs of Deficiency: Rickets, osteoporosis.
  Signs of Overdose: Deposits in body tissues, kidney stones, confusion, muscle pain.
  Supplement Needed? Yes.

CHLORIDE   *Estimated Minimum Daily Requirement (EMDR):* 750 mg (milligrams).
        Purpose: Helps maintain proper distribution and balance of body fluids, muscle and nerve function, digestion.
        Source: Normal salt intake, natural foods.
  Signs of Deficiency: Extremely rare; caused by illness, massive vomiting, or diarrhea.
  Signs of Overdose: Toxic in large amounts, but excess is excreted.
  Supplement Needed? No.

CHROMIUM   *EMDR:* 50–200 mcg (micrograms).
        Purpose: With insulin, regulates body's use of sugar; important to metabolism; may reduce risk of heart disease.
        Source: Lean meats, poultry, whole grains, eggs, cheese, brewer's yeast.
  Signs of Deficiency: Elevated blood sugar levels; diabetes-like symptoms such as poor muscle coordination, tingling in hands and feet.
  Signs of Overdose: If supplements with over 1,000 mcg used regularly, blocks insulin and can be toxic.
  Supplement Needed? Multinutrient supplement useful for most; not well absorbed.

COPPER   *EMDR:* 1.5–3 mg (milligrams).
        Purpose: Helps form hemoglobin; assists absorption of iron and regulation of blood pressure and heart rate; may help prevent cardiovascular problems.
        Source: Seafood, organ meats, green vegetables, nuts, cocoa, copper-piped water.
  Signs of Deficiency: Essentially limited to inherited diseases that prevent absorption.
  Signs of Overdose: Nausea, vomiting, stomach and muscle pain.
  Supplement Needed? No.

FLUORIDE   *EMDR:* 1.5–4 mg (milligrams).
        Purpose: Necessary for healthy teeth and bones; helps form enamel, which protects against cavities and decay; fluoride toothpaste helpful, but fluoridated drinking water much more effective (it is not harmful).
        Source: Fluoridated drinking water, sardines, salmon, cheese, meat, tea.
  Signs of Deficiency: Tooth decay, cavities, weakened teeth.
  Signs of Overdose: Extremely large amounts can cause softening and discoloration

of teeth, brittle bones; small amount in drinking water has only positive and no negative effects.

Supplement Needed? Nursing babies and children who do not drink fluoridated water may need supplements, but only as prescribed by doctor or dentist.

IODINE

EMDR for Adults: 150 mcg (micrograms).

EMDR for Pregnant Women: 175 mcg.

Purpose: Prevents enlargement of the thyroid gland (goiter); supports nutrient metabolism, nerve and muscle function, physical and mental development.

Source: Vegetables from iodine-rich soil, seafood, kelp; iodized salt—more than half of all salt consumed in U.S. is iodized—provides total iodine needed.

Signs of Deficiency: Goiter, weight gain, hair loss, mental retardation.

Signs of Overdose: Rare. Excess excreted.

Supplement Needed? Pregnant women may need in order to get EMDR; necessary to prevent mental retardation and dwarfism in newborns.

IRON

RDA for Adults: 10 mg (milligrams).

RDA for Premenopausal Women: 15 mg.

RDA for Pregnant Women: 30 mg.

Purpose: Strengthens immune function, essential to manufacture of hemo-globin (the blood substance that carries oxygen) and myoglobin (the substance that stores oxygen in muscles).

Source: Red meat, chicken, seafood, other animal products; dark green vegetables, nuts, whole grains. Breads and other foods are forti-fied with iron.

Signs of Deficiency: Fatigue, dizziness, heart palpitations, weakened immune func-tion; iron deficiency anemia.

Signs of Overdose: Vomiting, dizziness, fatigue. Overdose interferes with immune function and may increase risk of cancer or heart attack.

Supplement Needed? On M.D. recommendation can take multipurpose vitamin supple-ment. Never give children adult iron supplements, which can poison them.

MAGNESIUM

RDA for Women: 280 mg (milligrams).

RDA for Pregnant Women: 320 mg.

RDA for Men: 350 mg.

Purpose: Helps form and maintain bones and teeth; reduces risk of osteo-porosis; with calcium, regulates muscle activity; builds protein and converts food to energy; protects body against disease.

Source: Whole grains, fish, nuts, leafy green vegetables, milk.

Signs of Deficiency: Vomiting, muscle weakness, heart palpitations, tremor. Deficiency rare.

Signs of Overdose: Fatigue, muscle weakness.

Supplement Needed? No—kidneys conserve, excess is excreted; deficiency and toxicity are rare.

MANGANESE
EMDR: 2.5–5 mg (milligrams).
Purpose: Necessary for formation and maintenance of bone, cartilage, and connective tissues. Helps synthesize proteins and genetic material, produce energy from food, and assist blood clotting.
Source: Bran, bananas, strawberries, brown rice, whole grains, peas, beans.
Signs of Deficiency: Unknown. Deficiency rare.
Signs of Overdose: Unknown. Not toxic.
Supplement Needed? No. Diet easily provides needed amount.

MOLYBDENUM
EMDR: 75–250 mcg (micrograms).
Purpose: An enzyme component essential to development of nervous system; helps process waste; produces energy; mobilizes stored iron; detoxifies sulfites (food preservatives).
Source: Cereals, pasta, beans, milk, organ meats, leafy vegetables.
Signs of Deficiency: Deficiency not known to occur.
Signs of Overdose: Rare; continued use of molybdenum picolinate supplements at over 10 mg per day can cause joint pain and swelling.
Supplement Needed? No.

PHOSPHORUS
RDA for Adults over Age 25: 800 mg (milligrams).
RDA for Young Adults and Pregnant Women: 1,200 mg.
Purpose: Found in every cell, is essential for bone formation, bone, and teeth maintenance; helps muscle contraction and tissue repair, heart and kidney function.
Source: Almost all foods.
Signs of Deficiency: Deficiency rare, but may be caused by long-term use of antacids or other drugs containing aluminum hydroxide.
Signs of Overdose: Calcium loss; weak bones.
Supplement Needed? No.

POTASSIUM
EMDR: 2,000 mg (milligrams).
Purpose: Except for calcium and phosphorus, the body contains more potassium than any other mineral. With sodium and chloride, it assists nerve impulse transmission, muscle contractions, regulation of heartbeat and blood pressure; is required for proper function of protein, carbohydrate, and insulin secretion. May protect against heart problems, stroke, and high blood pressure.
Source: Raw vegetables, fruit, lean meats, and potatoes.
Signs of Deficiency: Severe deficiency: vomiting, diarrhea, muscle weakness and cramps, and abnormal heartbeat.
Signs of Overdose: Similar to signs of deficiency. Rare.
Supplement Needed? Yes, for those who do not get adequate amounts in diet.

SELENIUM
RDA for Women: 55 mcg (micrograms); future research may result in increased RDA.
RDA for Pregnant Women: 65 mcg
RDA for Men: 70 mcg

Purpose: Its antioxidant activity protects against free radicals; vitamin E and selenium mutually reinforcing; assists immune function; may help prevent arthritis, heart disease, and cancer.

Source: Mushrooms, whole grains, eggs, garlic, lean meats, and seafood.

Signs of Deficiency: Severe deficiency: vomiting, diarrhea, muscle weakness and cramps, abnormal heartbeat, nail and tooth problems.

Signs of Overdose: Toxic in high doses: hair loss, tooth decay, swelling in limbs.

Supplement Needed? No, diet typically provides the small amounts needed.

SODIUM

EMDR: 500 mcg (micrograms).

Purpose: Found in all body fluids, including blood, sweat, and tears; helps manage fluid distribution and balance, control muscle contraction, and regulate nerve function.

Source: Table salt, processed foods, meats, shellfish, soft drinks.

Signs of Deficiency: Too much, not too little, is problem in U.S.; temporary deficiency may occur with heatstroke.

Signs of Overdose: Body retains water, loses potassium; blood pressure increases.

Supplement Needed? No.

SULPHUR

RDA, EMDR: Not established.

Purpose: Every cell contains sulfur; with other vitamins, it assists metabolism, blood sugar regulation, blood clotting.

Source: Proteins: fish, meat, poultry, dairy products, beans, peas.

Signs of Deficiency: Deficiency does not occur in humans.

Signs of Overdose: Excess is excreted.

Supplement Needed? No.

ZINC

RDA for Adults: 15 mg (milligrams).

RDA for Pregnant Women: 30 mg.

Purpose: Synthesis of DNA and RNA requires zinc; contributes to numerous body processes including energy and cell metabolism.

Source: Lean meat, seafood, soybeans, peanuts, eggs, cheese, and wheat bran.

Signs of Deficiency: Loss of taste and appetite, hair loss, white streaks on nails, slow wound healing.

Signs of Overdose: Impaired immune function; vomiting, headaches, fatigue.

Supplement Needed? Multinutrient supplement may be needed, especially by young children, pregnant women, the elderly, and vegetarians.

9

Fasting and Juice Therapies

Fasting was practiced in many ancient cultures around the world but not typically in efforts to enhance health. Reasons for engaging in fasts included self-deprivation, political protest, demonstration of spiritual obedience, expression of grief, practicing cultural and religious ritual, and helping to generate hallucinations. Controlled, modified fasting under medical supervision also is used occasionally to help extremely obese people lose weight.

Fasting to achieve assumed health benefits, conversely, is a relatively recent phenomenon, practiced in prosperous Western societies. People do not practice health fasts in Bangladesh or Rwanda or third-world countries characterized by daily struggles for enough food to ward off starvation. Some view fasting for health-maintenance purposes as an affectation of affluence. Advocates see it as a route to internal cleansing and healing.

What It Is

Fasting involves restricting your dietary intake to a liquid. The liquid may be water, tea, or, most commonly today, vegetable or fruit juice. In the early 1990s, a juicing phenomenon swept the country. Juicers (Figure 9) were marketed widely and sold everywhere for prices ranging up to $500 and more. Juice bars were the rage, replaced more recently by *latte* and exotic coffee bars.

Proponents of fasting recommend occasional regular short fasts, lasting two to five days, as part of a general health-maintenance regimen. Advocates recommend that longer fasts for health maintenance or the healing of illness, lasting a month or more, be conducted under supervision at a fasting spa. For fasts lasting more than one week, juiced vegetables or fruits are given to supply the nutrients needed to maintain health. Some proponents add enemas as part of the detoxification fasting regimen.

What Practitioners Say It Does

Proponents claim that because the body is relieved of its usual chore of breaking food down into its elemental nutrients, fasting allows the body's inner resources to

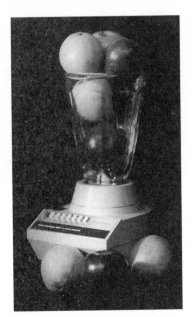

Figure 9 Fresh fruit juice is healthy as well as delicious, but juice fasts can be dangerous. The body needs more.

Dietary and Herbal Remedies

79

focus on cleansing and healing. Cleansing is said to be accomplished through the elimination of existing toxins.

Another major claim is that fasting enhances the immune system and reduces the demands placed on it. In addition to its role as part of health maintenance, some believe that fasting is an effective way to treat illnesses, including arthritis, ulcers, heart disease, asthma, and other problems.

Beliefs on Which It Is Based

The ancient belief that fasting purifies the soul has been extended to the current view that fasting can purify the body as well. The basic premise is that fasting maintains and restores health through physiological mechanisms. Included in these mechanisms, proponents claim, are shifting physiological effort from food conversion to the elimination of toxins, reducing the immune system's workload, releasing pesticides and other chemicals from body fat, and ridding the body of nonessential tissue.

It is helpful to look at these beliefs in terms of scientific information about the well-studied sequence of events that occurs when people start fasting. When body weight declines, water and fat—but not toxins—are lost from cells. Toxins are left behind.

Nutrients are needed to sustain immune competence, the ability of the body's disease-fighting immune system to make antibodies and other proteins and cells. Immune system failure, not enhancement, occurs when people do not eat enough to provide the nutrients that sustain proper immune function. Instead of reducing its workload, fasting impedes the immune system.

Proponents explain that people feel sick when fasting because toxins are leaving the body. Actually, fasting decreases the immune system's ability to destroy and eliminate toxins. Fasting also causes a drop in blood sugar levels, which causes a breakdown of tissues needed for energy. This leads people to feel sick because the brain and other tissues fail to receive needed sugars, and the body's metabolism is forced to remove the needed nutrients from muscle and liver tissue. At the same time, the liver and kidneys are not able to do their work of handling the by-products of protein breakdown.

Fasting can harm all organs. It is extremely dangerous to health, especially for those who are malnourished by chronic illness, yet some proponents recommend fasting to treat chronic illnesses. The slimmer the individual, the more dangerous a fast will be. The longer the fast, the more life-threatening it becomes. Studies show that when people reach 56 percent of their appropriate body weight, death occurs. The body cannot distinguish between intentional fasting and starvation.

Research Evidence to Date

Solid scientific research does not support the claims of fasting advocates. To the contrary, it contradicts those claims and indicates the dangers of fasting, even with water or juices. Reducing the number of calories you eat while maintaining a normal, balanced diet will reduce your weight. But consuming only water, tea, or juice is harmful, not helpful, to health and should be avoided especially by those who are ill.

What It Can Do for You

Proponents indicate that fasting can produce fatigue, anemia, irregular heartbeat, body aches, nausea, dizziness, and other negative effects. They refer to these as temporary problems that precede feelings of well-being, mental clarity, internal cleanliness, and other benefits.

Contrary to advocacy claims, fasting does not and cannot heal medical conditions, assist immune or other physiological function, or play a role in health maintenance. Even the hoped-for spiritual benefits of fasting—reducing your emphasis on bodily concerns—are questionable. The decreased supply of blood glucose leads the body to break down muscle for energy, causing weakness, depression, fatigue, and sick feelings. Depending on the individual, these reactions can begin as soon as the second day of a fast. Because the fasting individual feels weak and unwell, he or she tends to focus more attention on the body, not less.

10
Flower Remedies

Who among us has not experienced the therapeutic benefits of flowers—The delight of a field of wildflowers, the calming scent of a gardenia, the comfort of a bouquet? One man saw even greater power in flowers' ability to heal, and he created medications of their distillates.

In the early 1900s, the homeopathic English physician Edward Bach (pronounced to rhyme with "haitch") developed the theory that successful treatment of stress and negative emotions can heal physical disorders. He believed that physical treatment of the body alone can only "superficially repair" the damage caused by accident or disease. This is so, he explained, because "behind all disease lies our fears, our anxieties, our greed, our likes and dislikes." That is, illness is caused by underlying emotional problems or disorders. If a therapy could dispel unhappiness, distress, or other such difficulties, illness would disappear and people would be well. "Flower remedies" were developed to accomplish this goal.

Bach began studying the many varieties of flowers seen on his long walks in the English meadows and woodlands, eventually compiling a list of thirty-eight different therapeutic flowers. These were the blossoms found by Bach to cure various physical illnesses

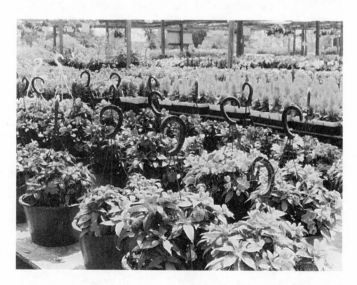

Figure 10 Flowers may not cure disease, but they elevate the spirit.

The Alternative Medicine Handbook

indirectly by eliminating the patient's emotional strife.

Following testing, particular flowers were specified as best for dealing with the seven categories of psychological disequilibrium that Bach identified: fear, uncertainty, general disinterest, loneliness, oversensitivity, despondency, and what he termed "over-concern for others." In addition to cures for each of these problem areas, he created a special group of five flowers to be used as a "rescue remedy" in crisis situations.

What It Is

Flower remedies are essences of flowers diluted in water and brandy. Drops of the preparation are placed directly under the tongue or in a glass of water or juice.

Those who use flower remedies focus on the perceived emotional cause of disease rather than the resultant disease itself. It is believed, for example, that a person suffering from diabetes (a result) has at the same time an underlying emotional or psychological problem (the cause of the illness, in this case diabetes).

The key is to define that person's emotional dysfunction. Once it has been identified, the proper flower remedy is pursued according to Bach's listings. Presumably, the negative emotion disappears, and with it goes the physical illness, whatever it happens to be. The particular physical ailment is not relevant to the treatment.

What Practitioners Say It Does

The flower remedies determined by Bach to treat a full range of ills are said to produce subtle, nontoxic results in varying lengths of time, depending on the severity of the problem. The remedies stabilize emotions and promote a general sense of well-being, stimulating an internal healing process. Some practitioners believe that flower remedies used in conjunction with other approaches, such as chiropractic manipulation, produce an even greater health-enhancing effect.

Beliefs on Which It Is Based

Bach concluded that flowers create "mechanisms" that forge links between the brain and the body, enabling the resolution of emotional problems and thereby curing the physical illness. The specific flower remedy to be

Producing Flower Remedies

Using Bach's method, flowers are picked in the early morning when they are in full bloom. Then they are soaked in unfiltered spring water while exposed to sunlight. After three hours, the blossoms are removed using a twig from the same flowering plant.

The fragrant water is then placed in a sterile bottle and mixed with an equal amount of brandy, creating a "mother essence." This liquid is diluted to create the remedy potion. Dilution follows homeopathic principles, meaning that very small amounts of the mother essence remain in the final remedy to be consumed.

Bach's Categories of Emotional Problems and Examples of Their Flower Remedies

1. **Fear** *Rock Rose* for terror, panic, fright, and nightmares; *Cherry Plum* for an inclination to uncontrollable rages and impulses, suicidal tendencies, or losing one's temper; *Aspen* for vague fears and anxieties of unknown origin or a sense of foreboding.

2. **Uncertainty** *Cerato* for doubting one's ability to make decisions; *Gentian* when even small delays cause hesitation, despondency, and self-doubt; *Gorse* for feelings of despair, hopelessness, and futility.

3. **Insufficient Interest in Present Circumstances** *Honeysuckle* for nostalgia, homesickness, and dwelling too much in the past; *Wild Rose* for apathy or making little effort to find joy; *Olive* for mental and physical exhaustion and sapped vitality; *Mustard* for sudden deep gloom that arises for no apparent reason.

4. **Loneliness** *Water Violet* for preferring to be alone, and for being aloof or reserved; *Impatiens* for impatience and feeling irritated by slower others; *Heather* for the self-absorbed who burden others with their troubles and dislike being alone.

5. **Oversensitivity to Influences and Ideas** *Centaury* for difficulty saying no and neglecting one's own interests; *Walnut* for stabilizing emotions during life transitions such as adolescence and menopause, for breaking past links and adjusting to new beginnings; *Holly* for envy, suspicion, revenge, and hatred.

6. **Despair** *Pine* for feeling self-reproach, guilt, and dissatisfaction with one's self; *Elm* for being overextended, for feeling overwhelmed with one's responsibilities; *Willow* for feeling life has treated one unfairly, for feeling resentful and unappreciated.

7. **Relationship Problems** *Chicory* for being possessive of others, demanding, and self-pitying, for needing others to conform to one's ideals; *Vine* for being autocratic, dictatorial, and ruthless; *Beech* for desiring perfection and easily finding fault with others.

---

applied in each case is determined by an evaluation of the patient's emotional state. Because the underlying emotional state is presumed to cause disease, the particular illness is not considered relevant when selecting the flower remedy.

Research Evidence to Date

Although no scientific evidence supports the idea that highly distilled floral essences can cure disease, Bach and his followers have collected scores of anecdotal reports. Many of these success stories are published as "Professional Testimonies" and "Emergencies: Professional Use" in a paperback book entitled *Bach Flower Remedies to the Rescue* by Gregory Vlamis (Healing Arts Press, Rochester, Vt., 1990). Here, flower remedies are reported not only for humans but also for animals. Testimonies from a range of health professionals and from consumers are reported.

Almost all of those who claim flower remedies as a means of curing illness emphasize their ability to work on "underlying emotional stress." In this sense, Bach was a pioneer in describing the important mind-body influences known today.

Scientific information about the mechanisms of mind-body action emerged decades after his death. Emotional states in many people can influence their physical well-being. Depression can lower immune function and leave the individual more vulnerable to illness in some instances. The subtle effect of flower remedies is thus said to attack the underlying problem of disease—emotional stress—mobilizing your own individual healing capabilities to promote a curative effect.

What It Can Do for You

Advocates suggest that the variety of flower remedies available today can help some people improve their sleep, reduce stress, calm fears, ease childbirth, reduce alcoholic tremors, and lessen skeletal and muscular pain. There are no scientific studies to support these claims, but flower remedies may evoke a placebo response. Flower remedies do not cure disease. As long as they are not used in place of needed professional care, they cause no harm and may provide a pleasant antidote to emotional stress.

Where to Get It

✦ Flower remedies are not widely used, and therefore tend to be rarely available in health-food stores.

✦ Ellon USA, formerly Ellon Bach USA, is credited with introducing the Bach flower remedies to the United States on a large scale. They will provide information by mail or phone: 644 Merrick Road, Lynbrook, NY 11563 (516 593-2206).

✦ Flower essences are sold by Pegasus Products, Inc., in Boulder, Colorado (303 667-3019), and Perelandra, Ltd., located in Warrenton, Virginia (703 937-2153).

✦ The Flower Essence Society in Nevada City, California (916 263-9162) distributes flower essences and imports herbs. The society maintains a full line of the thirty-eight flowers used by Bach.

Flowers Express and Evoke Emotion

Today as in ancient times, people use flowers to symbolize sentiments, bring out emotions, and express feelings. Although we may not drink floral essences to promote healing, we do bring flowers to the ill and injured to speed their recovery.

We give flowers to express and promote love and caring on special occasions such as anniversaries, graduations, and birthdays. Flowers beautify and sanctify weddings. They say hello and good-bye and help us to celebrate birth and mourn death. Particular flowers for Christmas and Easter are traditional holiday features.

We honor men and women of achievement with floral bouquets. Flowers are used to celebrate victories—the Kentucky Derby is called "The Run for the Roses"—and we drape the winner of the Indianapolis 500 in a wreath of blossoms.

11 ⁓
Herbal Medicine

Vinca rosea, a variety of the periwinkle plant, grows bright pink on the East Indian island of Madagascar. It has long been used there as an herbal remedy for diabetes. The periwinkle was brought to North America for scientific study in the late 1940s, and researchers in Canada and the United States identified its chemical structure. When a promising component of the plant was found to destroy cancer cells in a test tube, it was subjected to further study in animals. As in the test tube, the animals' cancers disappeared. Eventually, two forms of this chemical substance, vinblastine and vincristine, were approved for use against human cancers. They are still used today. Vinblastine attacks Hodgkins disease and many other cancers, and vincristine helps cure childhood leukemia and is used also to treat many types of cancer in adults. The plant has no role in the management of diabetes.

The Madagascar periwinkle plant story illustrates some of the blind alleys (diabetes) and rewards (cancer) of herbal medicine. It also clarifies the ongoing debate between herbalists who urge the medical use of plants as they grow in nature and other researchers who stress the importance of identifying and isolating their active components.

What It Is

Herbs are plants or plant parts, such as flowers, leaves, stems, bark, and roots, that are used to season foods (culinary herbs) or applied against health problems (medicinal herbs). Every culture throughout history has used plants to treat medical problems. Originally, the specific utility of herbs was assumed to be based on their shape or color. With this primitive **Doctrine of Signatures** approach, heart-shaped leaves were used against heart problems, plants with red flowers were applied to treat bleeding disorders, and so on.

However, the biological effects of herbs are due to their chemical ingredients, not their shape or color. Herbal remedies differ from prescribed pharmaceuticals in several ways. Typically, they include the entire herb

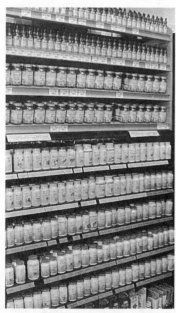

Figure 11 Increasing numbers of medicinal herbs are readily available.

or an entire part of the herb, such as the leaf. In contrast, pharmaceuticals, including those made from herbs, contain only the isolated and purified chemicals found to be the active ingredients, plus an inert liquid for tinctures or a binding substance for pills.

In North America and elsewhere, herbs are self-prescribed: we decide on our own to buy them (Figure 11). In Asia and some other parts of the world, herbal medicines frequently are prescribed by doctors. In either event, according to standard definitions of the term, herbal remedies are **drugs**, that is, substances used to treat an ailment or an illness. Herbs are much more dilute than the concentrated products we purchase in the local pharmacy, and they contain many more ingredients than do pharmaceuticals.

The best use for each medicinal herb was determined on a trial-and-error basis over time. This process of discovery no doubt caused many fatalities even as it documented positive results, because many herbs contain poisonous ingredients or substances that neutralize the main ingredient for which people take it. Today, **pharmacognosy** (the study of the biochemical aspects of natural products) works from the knowledge that "natural" does not necessarily mean "safe," and that raw herbs vary greatly in strength. Pharmacognosy seeks to standardize herbal products so that they consistently include the same amounts of active ingredients and are free of any harmful components that the plant may contain.

Each herb may hold many active chemical ingredients, and a single herb may harbor some helpful and some dangerous chemicals at the same time. Further, a particular chemical may be therapeutic in one amount and deadly in a slightly larger amount. This is the case with the foxglove plant from which digitalis is derived. Digitalis is an important drug used to treat heart failure. But slightly more than the therapeutic amount is fatal, as is consumption of the first-year's leaf growth of this plant.

More than one-fourth of conventional pharmaceuticals come from herbs. Sometimes a chemical isolated from an herb is copied in the laboratory so that the supply of the naturally growing plant is not threatened. Pharmaceuticals typically contain one active chemical

Caution

In the United States, we tend not to worry or even think much about the safety of the foods and drugs we buy. Nonprescription (over-the-counter) drugs, as well as prescribed pharmaceuticals, contain warnings, lists of possible side effects, and cautions about drug–drug interactions.

Behind these safety measures is careful evaluation by the FDA, which requires that all foods and drugs meet safety and quality standards. Herbal products do not fall under FDA jurisdiction. Therefore:

- Labels on herbal products rarely include information about risks, side effects, and possible harmful interactions with other substances.
- Herbal products may contain impurities, foreign objects, or highly varied quantities of the active ingredient you are paying for.
- Check with your doctor before using an herbal product, especially if you are taking any medications.
- Select herbs from reputable companies.
- Of greatest importance, do not use herbs for serious or potentially serious medical problems.

ingredient, tested and shown to be pure and effective.

Herbs are sold as dried or powdered remnants of the entire plant, the plant's active part, or as several plants mixed together. Herbal remedies usually contain many active ingredients. Herbs also can be purchased fresh, dissolved in a liquid, or in capsule form.

Medicinal herbs are not reviewed by the Food and Drug Administration (FDA) for safety and effectiveness. Legislation supported by the health-food industry, passed in 1994, took away the FDA's authority to test or preapprove dietary supplements such as herbs and vitamins.

Prior to that date, FDA reviews of safety and efficacy resulted in the elimination of many herbal ingredients in over-the-counter medications. These products are currently available, but now they lack FDA review and approval. Such review is required for all other over-the-counter (OTC) remedies, which cannot be marketed until they are standardized, proven safe and effective, and accurately labeled.

Many proponents and marketers fight to maintain the status quo of their OTC herbal remedies. They are unwilling to threaten their more than $1-billion-a-year business with FDA reviews of herbs for safety and effectiveness.

Others feel the public deserves better protection as well as information about useless products or harmful side effects. Such information typically is absent from herbal remedy packaging, sometimes because the herb has not been studied, so information about its effectiveness and side effects is unavailable.

What Practitioners Say It Does

Practitioners of herbal medicine indicate that herbs can be excellent alternatives to OTC medications or other home remedies. The general rule is that herbal remedies can be used safely and effectively for minor ailments that typically would be self-medicated. These ailments include minor aches and pains; stomach and digestive problems such as diarrhea; constipation and bloating; premenstrual syndrome (PMS), menstrual cramps, and cold cramps; colds and respiratory ailments; some arthritic, skin, and sleep difficulties; and other problems that people generally try to deal with themselves. Herbs should *not* be used for possibly serious medical problems, by pregnant women, or by people taking prescription medication.

Beliefs on Which It Is Based

Herbal products contain active chemical ingredients

Beware Unlikely Promises!
Blue-Green Algae Cancer Cure

In the 1980s, algae (a plant that lives primarily in water) from an Oregon lake was sold freeze-dried as a treatment for allergies, leprosy, arthritis, cancer, and other ailments. Similar products from other companies followed.

In addition to the fact that algae, dried or wet, is not known to be effective against any illness, government laboratory analyses found numerous additional and probably unwanted items in this product: parts of and whole maggots, ants, flies, insects, water fleas, and more.

Blue-green algae is popular again and available for sale.

The Potential Power of Herbal Ingredients

In the past ten years, more than 53,000 natural products were tested by the Natural Products Branch of the National Cancer Institute, including:

- 36,000 plants from twenty-five countries around the world
- 1,500 marine (water) plants
- 6,000 marine invertebrates
- 7,000 fungi and bacteria

Botanists work with local shamans to uncover potentially useful compounds, locating and screening in recent years approximately 10,000 natural compounds annually.

Scientists at the Natural Products Branch calculate that at least 40 percent of new drugs approved around the world between 1983 and 1994, including antibiotics, were derived from plant products, and more than half of the most important drugs prescribed in 1993 came from natural products.

Approximately one-third of all new cancer therapies come from a natural source. Examples include camptothecin, Taxol, cytosine arabinoside, and the AIDS drug AZT (azydothymidine).

The Story of Taxol

Since the 1950s, compounds from the bark of the Pacific yew tree have been believed to be beneficial:

1950–1960: The National Cancer Institute selects yew products for study and begins laboratory analyses.

1970s: The active ingredient is identified.

1979: The mechanism of action is uncovered.

1980s: Clinical trials document the chemical's safety, identify its side effects, and show its effectiveness in patients with ovarian cancer.

Late 1980s: Problem—use with patients is hampered because the chemical from the bark does not dissolve easily in water.

1993: Scientists synthesize Taxol from the natural product paclitaxel. In the process, they discover Taxotere (docetaxel), a potential analog of Taxol that eliminates the need to extract the chemical from the bark of the yew tree. Previously, extractions of 10,000 kg (kilograms) of bark, which destroyed 3,000 trees, had been necessary to obtain 1 kg of Taxol, enough to treat only 500 patients.

1994: An effective new cancer drug is available to treat patients.

that can have powerful effects on humans and other animals. In their natural state, herbs have been used to treat illness since antiquity, and in undeveloped areas of the globe, herbs still represent the main if not the only source of medicine. According to the World Health Organization (WHO), about 80 percent of people today must rely on traditional healing methods including herbal remedies, for care of illness.

Some proponents of medicinal herbs believe that a major benefit of natural herbs over manufactured pharmaceuticals is the collection of ingredients contained in medicinal herbs. Problems caused by one ingredient, they say, can be counterbalanced or neutralized by another.

This is correct in some cases but incorrect or unknown in others. Because medicinal herbs do not come with labels indicating which is which, trying an herb without investigating it first is like playing Russian roulette.

Research Evidence to Date

Many herbal remedies remain unstudied, and much of the research that has been conducted on medicinal herbs is not of the highest scientific quality. The herbal remedies listed below under "What It Can Do for You" represent only a small fraction of the medicinal herbs available in health-food stores, markets, and through the mail. They are included here because they are some of the safer and more popular products for self-use. Descriptions of the effectiveness and safety of these herbs is based on scientific research and commentary.

Because promotional material rarely includes information about toxicities, dangerous interactions, and other possible problems, consult your physician or an authoritative book before trying an herbal remedy. Many of the medicinal herbs described below are easily obtained or already stored in your kitchen as culinary herbs. The indications for use noted below have been scientifically substantiated.

What It Can Do for You

Aloe vera A soothing, healing skin gel contained in the leaf of the aloe vera plant. Many hand and body lotions and some cosmetics contain aloe. It is good for maintaining soft skin and to help heal sunburn and other minor surface burns, scrapes, and wounds. A small plant in a window of your home or office provides a fresh and ready supply: cut open a thick leaf and squeeze the liquid right onto your skin. The gel from inside the leaf should not be confused with the bitter yellow juice from the rind of the leaves. In dried form, this juice is a potent laxative.

Anise Tea made from crushed seeds of this licorice-flavored plant has been sipped since early Roman times to aid digestion and reduce nausea. Cough medications often contain anise.

Arnica Apply a cream containing chemicals from the herb arnica to treat burns and relieve acne.

Bearberry leaf For urinary tract infections, soak bearberry leaves in cold water overnight. Drink the strained liquid for no more than two days.

Blackberry, blueberry, or raspberry leaves To treat diarrhea, prepare tea by steeping 1-2 teaspoons of dried, finely chopped leaves in a cup of boiling water for ten minutes. Strain and drink.

Black cohosh extract The roots of this herb have been used to prepare medication for gynecologic disorders since ancient times. More recently, it was a major ingre-

Recommended References

Proponents and critics of herbal remedies alike recommend two books by herb expert and professor of pharmacognosy Dr. Varro Tyler: *The Honest Herbal: A Sensible Guide to the Use of Herbs and Related Remedies*, and *Herbs of Choice: The Therapeutic Use of Phytomedicinals* (both from Pharmaceutical Products Press, an imprint of Haworth Press, Binghamton, N.Y., 1993 and 1994, paperback).

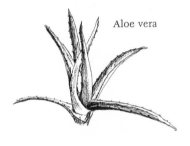
Aloe vera

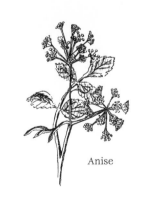
Anise

dient in Lydia Pinkham's popular remedy. The extract treats menopause problems, menstrual cramps and PMS. Do not use if pregnant: this herb has induced labor and caused birth defects in animals.

Blueberry fruit A tea made from dried blueberry fruit relieves diarrhea.

Bromelain Bromelain is an enzyme that reduces the kind of swelling and discoloration that can be caused, for example, by a sprain. Pineapples contain bromelain, but eating enough pineapple to do the job is likely to erode the inside of your mouth. Fortunately, bromelain is available in capsules.

Buckthorn bark Buckthorn is a relative of cascara (see below). A fluid extract works as an effective laxative.

Capsicum cream Apply for relief of muscle and joint aches. See cayenne—capsaicin is its active ingredient.

Cascara Over-the-counter medications for constipation contain compounds from this herb, which is an excellent laxative. Capsules of powdered bark are also available.

Cayenne The active ingredient in cayenne pepper, capsaicin, makes chili red hot. Capsaicin ointment applied to the skin relieves muscle aches and the joint pain of arthritis, and a new capsaicin product eases the inner-mouth sores sometimes caused by chemotherapy. The effect is produced by the chemical's ability to influence sensory nerve cells in the skin.

Chamomile Steeped for ten minutes in hot water, the daisylike flower of this plant produces a soothing tea that aids digestion and has a mild sedating effect.

Cinnamon Powdered cinnamon is more than a savory culinary herb. It can also help settle upset stomachs and relieve diarrhea, nausea, and vomiting.

Cranberry Cranberry juice may help ward off urinary-tract infections. See a doctor if the infection already exists; cranberry juice works only as a preventive measure.

Dandelion Tea brewed from dandelion root is cited often to treat digestion as well as liver, kidney, and bladder ailments. However, experts suspect that these remedies were founded in the Doctrine of Signatures (the yellow flower would be thought to treat yellow jaundice), and say there is no evidence of dandelion's medicinal

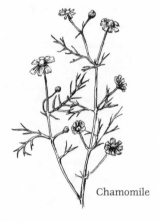

Chamomile

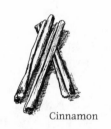

Cinnamon

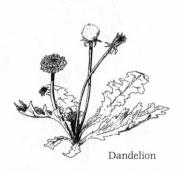

Dandelion

The Alternative Medicine Handbook

usefulness for these problems. Some believe that applying dandelion juice to warts can remove them.

Echinacea This well-studied plant helps treat infections through its ability to stimulate immune system activity. Tablets are used primarily to prevent and treat the common cold and related conditions such as sore throats.

Elderberry It may be only the soothing warm liquid or the inhaled steam, but hot elderberry tea is said to heal bronchitis and other problems of cold or flu.

English walnut leaves For skin rashes, boil the leaves in water, cool, strain, and apply to skin.

Ephedra (*Ma huang*) Danger! See the Warning box on page 97.

Eucalyptus For an effective cough remedy, drink freshly prepared tea made from eucalyptus leaves in water. Oil from the leaves is found in many nasal sprays, mouthwashes, ointments, and other products made to counteract the symptoms of colds and flu.

Feverfew Products that contain at least 2 percent parthenolide, feverfew's active ingredient, may well prevent and relieve migraine headaches and menstrual cramps.

Garlic Garlic is among the best studied of all medicinal herbs in history. Volumes of information document its effectiveness as a preventive and treatment for many problems. Whether fresh, dried, or commercially prepared, garlic's antibiotic action destroys fungal, viral, and bacterial infections. It helps prevent colds, flu, and other infections, and appears to work also as a chemopreventive, lowering the incidence of stomach cancer. Cardiovascular benefits include garlic's ability to lower high blood pressure, reduce blood cholesterol, and control excessive blood clotting.

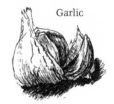

Garlic

Ginger Ginger tea aids digestion and soothes heartburn, and powdered ginger capsules, tea, or candy control motion sickness and nausea without causing drowsiness. Fresh ginger root relieves the sting of minor burns and can prevent and fight heartburn by absorbing stomach acid. A ginger compress can soothe carpel tunnel syndrome.

Ginkgo Extracts prepared from the leaves of the *Ginkgo* *biloba* tree appear to expand blood vessels, improve blood flow to the brain, and treat circulatory disorders and impotence. Used primarily to treat problems of the elderly, this serious medicine should be taken only under physician supervision.

Ginseng Commercial promotion has created the public image of ginseng as a wonder drug, capable of raising energy levels and modifying the effects of stress. There is no scientific evidence in support of these claims. Most American ginseng is exported *to* Asia, while most ginseng sold in the United States is imported *from* Asia. The amount of ginseng actually contained in commercial products available in the United States varies substantially, and some may contain no ginseng at all. An analysis of fifty-four ginseng products found that one-fourth contained none, and 60 percent contained only trace amounts of the herb. More information and better research are needed.

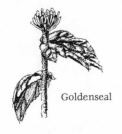
Goldenseal

Goldenseal The Cherokees and other Native American tribes have used this herbal remedy for centuries. As a tea it helps treat sores of the mouth and throat, and helps calm inflammations of the digestive and urinary tracts. A tea wash is a folk remedy for eye infections. Goldenseal contains berberine, an antibacterial chemical that lowers blood pressure and acts as a mild sedative.

Green tea Drinking at least one cup of green tea per week appears to reduce the risk of stomach cancer. Research on black tea, conversely, is contradictory, and further investigations are underway.

Horse chestnut Ointment made from the seeds of this herb may help reduce varicose veins.

Horseradish A taste of sauce made from its root opens the sinuses, and the plant helps destroy bacteria and fungi. Although the root has beneficial properties, the plant tops contain poisons known to be fatal to livestock.

Hypericum (St. John's wort) Possibly the most highly touted herbal remedy in recent U.S. history, this herb has long been popular in Europe as a primary treatment for mild to moderate depression. Experts believe that research underway in North America will substantiate the results of numerous European studies that document the effectiveness of this therapy. People on prescription medication for depression should not try hypericum without first talking with their physicians.

Iceland moss Tea brewed from this herb soothes the dry cough that often accompanies colds and flu.

Juniper Another herb with both culinary and medicinal value, juniper is used to flavor liquor and foods such as sauerkraut. Juniper tonic was used by Native Americans to relieve upset stomachs and cold symptoms, and as a diuretic. Diuretic action, which results from the plant's irritating effect on kidney tissues, expels fluid from the body in the urine.

Lavender oil Add some lavender oil to a warm tub and sink in for relaxation and relief of PMS. Parsley oil may accomplish the same goal.

Licorice Before it was learned that ulcers were caused by a bacterium, licorice was used to treat that condition. It is still considered useful as an expectorant and cough suppressant, and licorice lozenges and candies are used to treat common colds. Elderly persons and those with cardiovascular disease, liver, or kidney problems should be careful, because too much licorice can cause sodium retention, potassium excretion, and high blood pressure.

Ma huang **(ephedra)** Danger! See the box on page 97.

Milk thistle The seeds of this herb are said to help protect liver cells against antioxidants, but documentation is limited.

Nettle A tea made from the nettle root is an effective treatment for urinary difficulties related to benign prostatic hyperplasia (BPH), or enlarged prostate. It has minimal side effects. Dried leaves are often used as a diuretic to increase the flow of urine.

Oak bark Oak bark contains chemicals that work well as skin astringents and help heal rashes. Boil 2 teaspoons of powdered dried bark in a pint of water. Strain, cool, and apply to skin.

Parsley To freshen breath, chew fresh parsley.

Peppermint A widely used digestive aid, peppermint tea is a soothing, tasty brew that calms the stomach and may act as a mild sedative. Peppermint oil is popular in Europe to relieve severe skin itching. Peppermint tea treats diarrhea.

Juniper Can Be Toxic

Large or frequent doses of juniper cause kidney failure, convulsions, and digestive irritation.

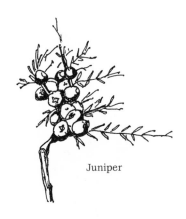
Juniper

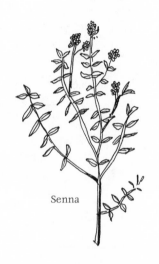

Senna

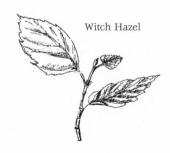

Witch Hazel

Plantago seed Also called "psyllium seed," this herb is an effective laxative. Take it with plenty of water.

Plantain Tea prepared with fresh or dried leaves will calm coughs and soothe the throat. It's helpful for colds and flu.

Saw palmetto Liquid extracts and tablets made from this shrub contain chemicals said to decrease the symptoms of benign prostatic hyperplasia (BPH), an enlarged but otherwise normal prostate gland. BPH commonly causes urinary-tract problems in men. However, research results are controversial. A 1995 review of the research from Germany concludes that saw palmetto and other herbal remedies for BPH are no better than placebos. The sale of saw palmetto preparations is forbidden in the United States.

Senna Senna is widely used as a laxative. Both syrup and tablets are marketed with FDA approval. Small leaves can be brewed in hot water or soaked in cold water for 12 hours to make tea. Prolonged use is associated with serious problems.

Slippery elm Consumed as a tea or in lozenges, used for coughs and minor throat irritations. Declared safe as an oral demulcent by the FDA.

Valerian This herb may be prepared as a tea or taken as an extract. It has well-documented calming effects. It works as a minor tranquilizer and as a sleep aid. It also relieves backache and other problems caused by tight muscles.

Volatile mustard oil Muscle aches and pains respond to brief application of diluted volatile mustard oil. The oil is extremely irritating and must be highly diluted to represent no more than 5 percent of the mustard plaster. Use a little in alcohol or in a flour and water paste. Leave on skin for less than ten minutes to avoid blistering. **Wintergreen oil** is used in a similar fashion.

Watercress Fresh leaves reduce fatigue and have been used traditionally as a diuretic and to treat rheumatism and bronchitis.

Witch hazel Applied to the skin to treat hemorrhoids, itching, and minor pain, the bottled witch hazel commonly found on drug store shelves helps bruises and

Warning: Herbal Products with Serious Toxic Effects

1. Products with ingredients that can produce serious harmful consequences:
   - Chaparral tea, from leaves and twigs of a desert shrub called the creosote bush, is promoted as an antioxidant, a pain reliever, and other uses. It has caused liver failure requiring liver transplantation.
   - Preparations such as some Indian herbal tonics that cause lead poisoning.
   - Herbs that counteract or enhance the activity of prescription medication for cardiac problems or bleeding disorder.
   - *Jin Bu Huan*, an ancient Chinese sedative and analgesic containing morphinelike substances, which causes hepatitis.
   - Chan su (topical aphrodisiac sold as "Stone," "LoveStone," "Rockhard") caused death when ingested.
   - Coltsfoot (for respiratory problems), comfrey (for arthritis, infections), and sassafras (a general tonic) caused liver problems and cancer in lab animals.
   - Kombucha tea, made from mushroom culture (used as a cure-all), caused deaths from acidosis.
   - Lobelia (used for respiratory congestion) caused respiratory system paralysis, and death.
   - Pennyroyal tea made from leaves treats coughs and upset stomach, but oil is highly toxic to liver and inhibits blood clotting.
   - Yohimbe bark (used as aphrodisiac) raises blood pressure and is associated with psychotic episodes.
   - Diet pills that contain ephedra (*ma huang*), a potentially deadly herb.
2. Products promoted as cures for illnesses they do not cure:
   - Essiac or mistletoe for cancer.
   - Pau D'Arco tea for cancer and AIDS.
3. Herbs sold to achieve street drug "legal highs" that cause heart attacks, seizures, psychotic episodes and death:
   - *Ma huang*, or ephedra, is an herbal form of the central nervous system stimulant commonly known as speed, sold with names like Herbal Ecstasy, Cloud 9, and Ultimate XPhoria.
4. Herbal products that are fake or highly contaminated :
   - In 1996, the Chinese government found widespread adulteration, contamination, illegal ingredients, and fake products in many of its herbal remedies. Illness and deaths resulted in China. The government closed most medicinal herb markets throughout China until new production guidelines could be established and enforced.
5. Products that contain something other than what is indicated on the label:
   - "Siberian ginseng" capsules may contain instead a weed full of male hormonelike chemicals.
6. Products based only on unverified, scanty, anecdotal evidence, sold by the promoter:
   - Cat's claw, or *una de gata*, from Peru.

swellings. The liquid also relieves cold sores, hives, oily skin, sunburn, poison ivy, and poison oak.

Where to Get It

Medicinal herbal products are available in capsule and liquid form in health-food stores and many shops and markets. Dried herbs individually and in combinations are sold in ethnic markets, but their potential for contamination and toxicity is high.

Because herbs, like other drugs, can be dangerous both by themselves or in certain combinations, caution is important. Consider these guidelines:

+ Check with an expert in botanical medicine.
+ Contact NAPRALERT (Natural Products Alert) for information about specific herbs from a database of 126,000 articles: College of Pharmacy-UIC, 833 South Wood Street, Chicago, IL 60612 (312 996-2246).
+ Consult an authoritative book such as Varro Tyler's *The Honest Herbal* (1992) or *Herbs of Choice* (1994) (both published by Haworth Press, New York), or Steven Foster and James Duke's *Medicinal Plants* (Houghton-Mifflin Company, Boston, 1990).
+ Read the comprehensive summary article about herbal products in the November 1995 issue of *Consumer Reports*.
+ Beware of some pop publications about herbal remedies. Many contain misinformation and incorrect data.
+ Contact the American Botanical Council in Austin, Texas (512 331-8868). They publish booklets about herbs as well as *HerbalGram* magazine.
+ Check with the Herb Research Foundation in Boulder, Colorado (303 449-2265).

Macrobiotics

Although a relatively recent creation, the macrobiotic diet is based in large part on the yin-yang principle of balance, a fundamental component of ancient Chinese medicine (see Chapter 3). Yin and yang are opposite forces believed to describe all components of life and the universe. Here the worldview of balance is embodied in diet, including the selection, preparation, and consumption of foods.

The macrobiotic diet was developed by George Ohsawa, a Japanese philosopher who sought to integrate traditional Asian medicine and belief with Christian teachings and some aspects of Western medicine. Starting in the 1930s, he taught a philosophy of healing through proper diet and natural medicine. He moved to Boston in 1960, where an early disciple, Michio Kushi, came to spearhead the macrobiotic way of life.

What It Is

The macrobiotic diet is more than a prescription for specific foods and their preparation. It is also a spiritual and social philosophy of living, plus a fully formed, unique concept of human physiology and disease. Because this concept was developed without benefit of professional training or knowledge of anatomy and physiology, it is fanciful and far from accurate. It states, for example, that blood cells, which actually are produced in the bone marrow, are birthed by a "mother red blood cell" in the stomach.

Macrobiotic "diagnostic techniques," including **iridology**, or looking at a person's eyes to diagnose cancer and other diseases (Figure 12), appear to be less commonly accepted than they were a few decades ago. This is fortunate because in the past many sick people failed to have their illnesses properly diagnosed, and they received proper treatment belatedly if at all, sometimes with fatal results. Also, some individuals were "diagnosed" with a cancer they did not really have, "cured" with macrobiotics, and presented publicly as evidence of the ability of macrobiotics to cure cancer. This kind of activity perpetuated an unfortunate cycle. Neither macrobiotics nor any other diet can cure cancer.

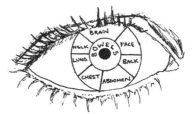

Figure 12 Iridology, a disproven diagnostic technique based on studying the iris of the eye, is used by some macrobiotic practitioners.

Dietary and Herbal Remedies

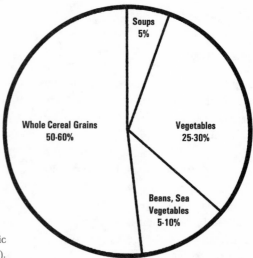

Figure 13 Pie chart of the standard macrobiotic diet (includes occasional supplementary foods).

Setting aside the philosophy, the erroneous beliefs about how the human body functions, and the useless diagnostic techniques, aspects of the diet itself have merit if not carried to extremes. You need not ascribe to or even think about the imaginary systems behind it. Initially the macrobiotic diet consisted almost exclusively of brown rice and a very limited amount of liquid. It was nutritionally deficient, causing a few deaths from starvation.

Later enhanced, it now derives 50 to 60 percent of its calories from whole grains, 25 to 30 percent from vegetables, and the remainder from beans, seaweed, and soups (Figure 13). Soups made with miso, which is a product of the fermentation of soybeans, remain an important dietary component. Soybean-based foods are encouraged in general, a small amount of fish is permitted, and processed foods are to be avoided.

In-season foods are preferred, and food is to be prepared in very specific ways. Vegetables, for example, should be cooked for long periods of time (a procedure that diminishes their nutritional value). Rice must be pressure-cooked. Only gas stoves are to be used, and utensils should be constructed of wood or other natural materials, glass, ceramic, enamel, or stainless steel. Copper pots, aluminum utensils, and electric stoves are to be avoided.

Foods Prohibited in the Macrobiotic Diet

· Coffee
· Dairy products
· Eggs
· Sugar
· Processed foods
· Meats

The Alternative Medicine Handbook

What Practitioners Say It Does

Proponents of the macrobiotic diet believe that it cures cancer, that it prevents illness, and that it promotes good health and harmony with the external world. The explanations given for these effects concern energy, vibrations, and yin-yang balance, all abstract notions that cannot be measured or even detected.

Beliefs on Which It Is Based

Within the yin-yang ideology, whole-grain foods (Figure 14) are considered ideal, not because they are low-fat, low-cholesterol, low-calorie, high-fiber foods, but because they are neutral: neither too yin (female) nor too yang (male).

Research Evidence to Date

There are three related but distinct areas of consideration regarding the macrobiotic diet: its philosophical context, the merits of the overall diet, and the value of particular ingredients. Each must be considered.

The philosophical context involves the idea of balancing foods that are yin and those that are yang, of calculating the yin or yangness of the season and of one's geographic location when selecting and preparing foods, and, for cancer patients, of balancing yin cancers with yang foods and vice versa. No research supports these mystical ideas. If eating certain foods evokes a desired closeness to nature or universal harmony, fine. But that is all one can expect from these ideas. They have no practical or therapeutic value.

The macrobiotic diet, however, can have value if not taken to extremes. The diet lowers fat and cholesterol in the body, reduces weight, and produces results associated with low-fat diets. These beneficial results include lower blood pressure and reduced chances of *getting* heart disease and certain cancers that appear related to fat intake, such as breast cancer.

Caution is crucial, however, because the diet can be seriously deficient in particular nutrients. In the past five years, several studies of the macrobiotic diet have been reported in the peer-reviewed medical literature. One concerned breast-feeding women, and the rest evaluated the diet for infants and children. The studies were

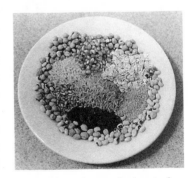

Figure 14 Grains are the heart of the macrobiotic diet (and of USDA recommendations).

conducted in Belgium, Norway, the Netherlands, Germany, and the United States.

Every study found serious deficiencies in infants and children who had been on macrobiotic diets. Problems in children included nutritional rickets with breathing abnormalities as well as bone deformities, vitamin B_{12} deficiency, growth retardation, deficiencies of protein, vitamins, calcium, and riboflavin, leading to retarded growth and slower psychomotor development. The study of lactating macrobiotic mothers mirrored these results, finding that the mothers' milk was deficient in essential vitamins. Researchers recommend that children on the macrobiotic diet receive dairy products and eggs to provide the missing nutritional components and produce a safer, balanced diet. Pregnant and breast-feeding women similarly should supplement their macrobiotic diets.

The third component of macrobiotic research concerns specific products or ingredients. Although no food products cure disease, the preventive benefits of some foods are well documented. Along these lines, scientists are investigating the potential anticancer properties of genistein, a substance in soybeans. Consumption of genistein through soybeans may be an explanation for Asian women's lower rates of breast and other cancers relative to those of American women. Soy versus animal protein has been shown in scientific studies to decrease cholesterol. The lower fat intake associated with dietary soy products may help decrease the incidence of breast cancer.

There are lessons to be drawn from the combination of positive and negative features of macrobiotics. First, there are no magic cures or even magic diets. Second, like the pearl in the oyster, something important and worthwhile may be hidden inside a shell of little value. Finally, the macrobiotic diet, like other vegetarian diets, requires supplementation to balance its deficiencies. A properly supplemented macrobiotic diet has benefits.

What It Can Do for You

A low-fat diet, high in grains, soup, and vegetables, supplemented with eggs, cheese, and fish to ensure adequate nutrition, plus plenty of liquid, can help prevent heart disease and some cancers and keep you slim and fit.

Where to Get It

Information about macrobiotics is available in health-food stores. Generally, however, these proponent books do not make mention of the cautions and supplements needed by special groups such as infants and children, the elderly, the seriously ill, and women who are pregnant or breast feeding.

Ingredients and recipes for healthful vegetarian diets, which may be seen as upgraded macrobiotic diets, are available in vegetarian cookbooks. Numerous excellent vegetarian cookbooks line the cookbook section shelves of most bookstores. One volume many find to be helpful is:

+ *The Wellness Encyclopedia of Food and Nutrition*, edited by Sheldon Margen and the Editors of the *UC Berkeley Wellness Letter* (Rebus, New York, 1992).

Caution

Even supplemented with the missing vitamins, calcium, and proteins, macrobiotic, and other diets with very low fat content may have too few calories for good health.

Caloric deficiencies may be harmful to people who expend a lot of energy, to infants and children, and to breast-feeding mothers.

13 🖎

Vegetarianism

People who eat plant products primarily or exclusively are called vegetarians. Eating only vegetables used to be considered an exotic or religious practice. The diets of Seventh-Day Adventists, Hindus (who revere and protect cows), 1960s commune enthusiasts, and most of the "underdeveloped world" exclude meat and rely on less expensive, more-available plant-grown food. As it turns out, the less expensive, plant-based diet, with some qualifications, is much more healthful than is the typical meat-oriented diet.

What It Is

Vegetarians may adopt several types of different diets:
- **Raw-food vegetarians** restrict their diet to only sprouted beans and sprouted grains in addition to raw vegetables and nuts. This most extreme diet excludes added fats, oils, salt, and all other flavorings.
- **Vegans**, or strict vegetarians, consume only food generated by plants. These foods include vegetables, fruits, grains, beans, and nuts.
- **Lactovegetarians** consume plant-based foods plus dairy products, including milk, butter, and cheese.
- **Lacto-ovovegetarians** add eggs to the lactovegetarian diet.

Many people develop their own vegetarian approach, adding fish to an otherwise vegan diet, or eating dairy products on occasion. Vegetarian diets may sound dull and dreary to people who have never tried them. Restaurants, magazine recipes, and cookbooks, however, display attractive and varied dishes that most people find tasty and satisfying. Vegetarian meals no longer are restricted to people in economic need or to cultural extremists.

What Practitioners Say It Does

Enthusiasts stress the health benefits of a balanced vegetarian diet. Balance is the operative and crucial concept because extremists can experience protein deficiencies serious enough to become a threat to health and life.

Careful!

Vitamin D and especially vitamin B_{12} deficiencies may occur with vegetarian diets.

The potential for B_{12} deficiency is of special concern in children and pregnant or lactating women.

B_{12} supplements or a daily general vitamin tablet are recommended.

The Alternative Medicine Handbook

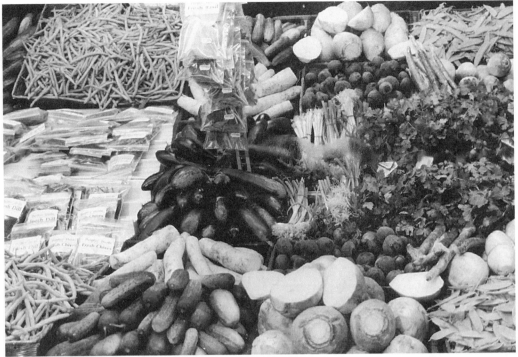

Figure 15 Fresh vegetables offer greater benefit than vitamin pills.

Protein is well named. It comes from a Greek word meaning "of prime importance." Protein is necessary not only to ensure energy, but for the very maintenance of life itself. It is essential to the metabolic activity of every cell. Combinations of whole-grain products (rice, breads, and corn tortillas) and legumes (beans, peas, and chick-peas), in a two-to-one ratio favoring grains provide the needed protein.

Beliefs on Which It Is Based

Varied convictions lie behind people's decisions to adopt full or partial vegetarian diets. Some believe that it is more natural for humankind to forego animal meats, as we lack the flesh-tearing teeth and short intestines of carnivorous animals, but share with vegetarian mammals the flat molars to grind plants and seeds and the long intestines needed to break down and absorb plant foods. Perhaps we did not evolve to become meat eaters.

Religious, cultural, or philosophical preferences to avoid animal products have propelled people in the

Enough Protein?

Westerners are accustomed to getting their protein from meat. Plant products, however, including vegetables, grains, and fruit, also contain protein. A balanced fruit-and-vegetable diet supplies enough protein to meet daily adult requirements.

Dietary and Herbal Remedies

Soy

High in protein, soy products also reduce LDL, the "bad" cholesterol, lower blood pressure, and seem to reduce night sweats and hot flashes often associated with menopause.

Western world away from animal products. Some view the slaughter of animals as cruel and immoral, as did those who founded the American Vegetarian Society in 1850. Those nineteenth-century reformers also maintained the ideology that meat consumption was immoral, calling meat a "stimulant."

Many are drawn today to the habits of early cultures that practiced a more aesthetic, vegetarian lifestyle. That such diets may have been imposed by ecological or economic necessity does not diminish their appeal.

Probably most people who switch to meatless fare today do so for their health—to lose weight, to reduce cholesterol and the risks of coronary artery disease, and possibly to help prevent some cancers—and these are compelling reasons.

Research Evidence to Date

Scientific research has documented the relationship between vegetarian diets with no or very low cholesterol and decreased risk of heart disease, diabetes, high blood pressure, obesity, and colon cancer. Plant-based foods contain no cholesterol. Cholesterol exists only in animal products. Strict vegetarian diets are free of cholesterol, but they are not free of fat.

Very small amounts of fat are essential to meet basic nutritional needs, and fat is found in most foods, including vegetables and grains. Not the presence, but the type of fat makes the difference. Animal products produce saturated fat, which increases cholesterol levels, while the fat contained in most vegetables is unsaturated. Unsaturated fat reduces cholesterol. Exceptions include avocados, coconuts, and tropical oils, all of which contain saturated fats.

What It Can Do for You

Total or partial, a well-balanced vegetarian diet is good for your health (Figure 15). Even cutting back on animal meats and full-fat dairy products helps, as does increasing your intake of fresh fruits and vegetables. Vegetarian diets also are less expensive.

If you now eat like the average American and want to move toward a more vegetarian diet, start gradually. Begin by reducing meat and changing to low- or no-fat dairy products. At the same time, introduce increased amounts of fiber-containing vegetables and grains gradually, so that your system has a chance to adjust.

Neither total nor extreme vegetarianism is necessary to experience health benefits. The recommended food pyramid put out by the USDA for daily diets (see the introduction to Part II) can be a good start or a very healthful goal.

Where to Get It

+ Information is available from the Vegetarian Resource Group, P.O. Box 1463, Baltimore, MD 21203, and the North American Vegetarian Society, P.O. Box 72, Dolgeville, NY 13329.
+ The Internet contains many Web sites about vegetarianism and about nutrition generally.
+ Vegetarian magazines may be useful: *Vegetarian Times* (800 435-9610); *Vegetarian Journal* published in Baltimore, Maryland (410 366-vege); *Veggie Life* published in Mt. Morris, Illinois (510 671-9852).
+ There are also newsletters, including *A Vegan's Journal*, P.O. Box 2552, Madison, WI 53701-2252; *Nutrition Advocate* (800 841-0444); *The Nutrition Action Health Letter* published by the Center for Science in the Public Interest, 1875 Connecticut Avenue NW, Suite 300, Washington, DC 20009-5728 (202 332-9111).
+ Numerous vegetarian cookbooks are available in libraries, health-food stores, and bookshops.

PART THREE

USING THE MIND FOR EMOTIONAL RELIEF AND PHYSICAL STRENGTH

Before medicine emerged from its religious and mystical roots, the mind was believed to play a major role in health. Centuries later, when bacteria and other scientific causes of disease were uncovered, the mind and body were separated in medical thinking, only to be merged again in recent decades.

The idea that our thoughts and emotions can affect our physical status has worked its way into our idioms with phrases such as "worry yourself sick," and "you're going to give yourself a heart attack." Can we really "worry ourselves sick?" Can the mind heal or cause illness, or at least ameliorate or aggravate symptoms? Early Greek practices, traditional Chinese medicine, Ayurvedic medicine, and virtually all ancient healing systems emphasize mind-body interactions.

Modern medicine reduced the emphasis on emotional and mental factors as a source of disease for two main reasons. First, many mind-based explanations of disease, unsupported by evidence, have been proven wrong: we have tended to attribute psychological or emotional causes to diseases such as tuberculosis and diabetes until their actual causes were discovered. Second, advances in fields such as microbiology, pathology, and molecular biology have uncovered many physical agents of disease, replacing old beliefs with new bacterial and genetic explanations. Gastric ulcers are a good example. Thought for decades to be caused by stress-produced acid, most ulcers are now known to be caused by the bacterium *Helicobacter pylori*. Such ulcers can be totally eradicated with a course of antibiotics, which kills the bacteria.

In the last few decades, however, research groups

have applied modern scientific methods to old mind-body questions, seeking to understand how thoughts, expectations, and emotions influence health. These investigators work in the area known as **mind-body medicine**, also called **behavioral medicine**. Behavioral medicine programs have been established at the most prestigious medical centers in the United States and in other countries. Investigators study meditation, hypnosis, biofeedback, and other previously esoteric activities for evidence about how the ancient wisdom concerning links between mind and body can be documented, explained, and applied to assist modern health care.

One of the first spurs toward mind-body medicine was a relatively simple discovery made in a doctor's office. When the first medication to reduce hypertension (high blood pressure) was developed, many patients taking this medication to lower blood pressure reported the opposite effect: their blood pressures increased. It turned out that the stress and anticipation of the visit to the doctor caused blood pressures to rise, a phenomenon dubbed "white-coat hypertension."

These initial insights, along with research on the physiological effects of stress, led mind-body medicine to focus much of its attention on how the body and mind respond to stressful situations, on how those responses affect our health, and on what, if anything, we can do to change our responses to stress.

Four basic questions are asked in assessing mind-body medicine. First, what is stress and what role does it play in illness? Second, what disorders can be influenced by mind-body techniques? Third, which mind-body techniques are available and usable? Finally, what are the possible pitfalls and benefits of the mind-body approach?

Stress is defined as a short-term reaction to a potentially threatening situation. Its evolutionary roots go back to the time when wild animals and other immediate threats to human existence demanded immediate, powerful reactions. When confronted with a threat or a perceived threat, the **autonomic nervous system** (the nervous system outside of our conscious control) mobilizes a whole group of organs into action, alerting and preparing the body to flee or confront the stressor. These organs work by releasing adrenaline and other hormones into the bloodstream. The reaction is known as the **fight-or-flight response**.

The problem comes when we are exposed to a continuing series of events that we perceive, even sometimes incorrectly, to be stressful. Many researchers believe that the perception of chronic stress is what causes deleterious physiological results, such as a weakening of the immune system or the aggravation of symptoms associated with an existing condition. With chronic stress, the hormonal and physiological changes caused by the fight-or-flight response become frequent and prolonged, creating an environment in which illness can more readily occur.

There are two main puzzles associated with the evaluation of stress. First, life's misfortunes, from minor snubs to major tragedies such as the death of a loved one, are fairly obvious causes of stress. However, research evidence shows that seemingly positive events, such as marriage, a shift to a better job, a new baby, and so on, also can act as stressors. Indeed, the process of change in and of itself appears to induce stress. Second, the perception of stress varies markedly from one person to the next, based on temperament and genetic predisposition. Some thrive on situations that, in other people, cause serious emotional problems or paralysis of will.

It seems plausible on the surface that stress should or could cause disease, and this idea certainly has found a place in our folklore. But what evidence shows that stress or emotions do indeed play a role, if not to cause disease, then at least to aggravate its symptoms?

For the two leading causes of death in America—cancer and heart disease—the evidence has been mixed. There seems to be little evidence supporting the idea that stress plays a major role in the development or progression of cancer. Genetic, environmental, and behavioral factors such as smoking, obesity, and inactivity seem to play the primary etiologic or causal roles.

However, stress appears to be an important contributing factor in the development of heart disease. Furthermore, many other problems such as chronic pain, diabetes, arthritis, asthma, and skin conditions have major psychosomatic characteristics, and thus may be caused in part by stress, or, more likely, have their symptoms exacerbated by stress.

In the past few years alone, a rash of solid scientific studies have shown the following: that depression predicts cardiac death within eighteen months (Montreal Heart Institute); that emotional stress predicts heart problems better than the commonly used exercise stress test and may actually initiate heart disease (Duke University and collaborating medical centers); that there is a strong association between anxiety and increased risk of sudden cardiac death (Harvard University); that depression and hopelessness play a role in heart disease (Centers for Disease Control and Prevention); and additional similar data.

Mind-body approaches may offer substantive hope. If mind-body techniques can reduce perceived levels of stress, depression, anxiety, and other chronic negative reactions, some serious illness could be avoided. Quality of life for those who suffer from disorders of anxiety or depression could be greatly enhanced.

Theoretically, any method that could alleviate or counteract the effects of stress should improve our health. What are the mind-body approaches, and can they accomplish this goal? The predominant approaches involve efforts to train either the mind, through activities like meditation and biofeedback, or the body, through programs such as yoga and exercise. The chapters in this part deal with the former set of efforts.

The various mind-body approaches have two things in common: they are systematic methods involving practice and discipline, and their physiological effects are documented and correlated with an increased ability to manage stress. Meditation involves focusing attention on an object or mental picture over a period of time. It is a foundation of mind-body medicine research, based on discovery and analysis of the relaxation response. Researchers found that brief (fifteen to twenty minute) periods of sitting still and concentrating on breathing, while reciting a word with each breath, lowered blood pressure, decreased heart rate, and decreased galvanic skin response (a measure of stress). Meditation is an integral component of the world's major religions, as it is of ancient healing systems.

Biofeedback involves the use of a machine to monitor functions such as heart rate, muscle tension, pulse, or breathing rate. By consciously seeking to alter these body functions through gauging the changes produced, one can learn to regulate physiological activity to a degree. The other mind-body techniques discussed in this part, such as hypnosis and imagery, accomplish the same goal—relaxation—but without the use of equipment.

The mind-body thesis is a seductive explanation of illness, giving patients a sense of control or allowing others to cite patients' behavior as the reason for their illnesses. Although chronic negative emotions appear to play a role in the development of heart disease and other illnesses, it is not always a major role. In cancer it is likely that prolonged stress, anger, or other negative mental states represent but one link in a long causal or explanatory chain. Many mental illnesses, such as schizophrenia, and some forms of substance abuse that were thought to be defects of character, are now linked to complicated sets of defects and imbalances in brain chemistry.

When reasoning or research show a general correlation between a disease and a measure of mind-body health, it does not mean that a particular patient's illness is caused by improper or inadequate attitude. The main benefits of mind-body therapies are attained through their ability to effectively reduce stress. These benefits include illness prevention in specific cases and symptom relief—which typically are low-cost, self-administered, and free of side effects.

Thirty years ago the Western world discovered what had been known for a thousand years in the East: people who can identify their own physiological responses, such as changes in skin temperature, blood pressure, and brain-wave activity, also can learn to control those responses. Controlling and changing physiological activity is possible through mental effort, sometimes accompanied by physical activity such as regulated breathing or altered posture. Technology that illustrates the mechanisms of mind-body processes by making them visible or audible—thus providing feedback about the internal events—facilitates this effort.

As a result of this amazing discovery, and concurrent with the development of increasingly sophisticated devices to measure and record bodily activity of all types, scientific and public interest grew. Biofeedback (*bio* meaning "life") came to be seen as an exciting new therapeutic tool. Applications of the biofeedback technique have been continually developed to address various physical problems.

What It Is

Biofeedback is a mind-body process that uses monitoring equipment to provide visual or audible signs of muscle and autonomic nervous system activity. These internal changes can be viewed on computer screens, or information about them can be provided by sounds that vary in pitch as physiological variation occurs. Instrument readings that measure muscle tension, skin temperature, perspiration, pulse rate, and breathing allow patients to observe any changes that result from their behavior or thought processes. In time, patients can learn to modify the targeted physiological activity.

The five most common kinds of biofeedback are electromyographic, thermal, electrodermal, finger-pulse, and respiration.

Electromyography (EMG) measures muscle tension and is used to treat muscle stiffness, chronic muscle pain, and incontinence. It is applied also for physical rehabilitation of injured muscles.

Thermal biofeedback measures the temperature of the skin, which provides an index of blood-flow change. It can relieve hypertension, migraine headaches, anxiety, and Raynaud's disease (a circulatory condition that keeps the fingers and toes abnormally cold).

Electrodermal activity (EDA) measures changes in perspiration that are otherwise too minor to detect. Electrodermal feedback is often applied to treat anxiety.

Finger pulse feedback measures both pulse rate and amount of blood in each pulse. Hypertension and anxiety, as well as cardiac arrhythmias, can be controlled with finger-pulse measurements.

In **respiration feedback**, monitors measure the rate, volume, and rhythm of the patient's breathing, and determine whether the individual is using chest or abdominal breathing. These breathing measurements can help alleviate problems of hyperventilation, asthma, and anxiety. Learning breath control can contribute to enhanced relaxation in general.

In a typical biofeedback session, electrodes leading from a monitoring machine are attached to the part of the body to be monitored, such as muscles, head, hands, fingers, or feet. The monitoring device produces a variable-pitch tone or a visual readout, reflecting activity

---

Using Biofeedback versus Meditation

Biofeedback is a relatively modern mind-body technique involving the use of computers to display body functions such as heart rate. Monitoring these activities at various levels enables people to observe how and why they change and eventually to control them.

The ability to gain control over what had been considered to be involuntary or autonomic physiological functions was documented in biofeedback studies in the 1970s. However, since ancient times, practitioners of yoga and Zen Buddhism have achieved similar control using meditation without the benefit of modern monitoring equipment.

Meditation involves resting quietly and performing mental exercises to achieve a state of profound relaxation and focused concentration.

Electroencephalogram (EEG) studies of yoga and meditation confirmed parctitioners' ability to produce changes in brain-wave activity. It has been shown that, with meditation and concentration alone, people can lower their blood pressure, heartbeat, and respiration; reduce their oxygen consumption and blood lactate levels; and change other internal activities.

---

detected at the electrode contact points on the patient's body.

A biofeedback therapist helps interpret these signals while leading the patient through physical and mental exercises, attempting to produce changes in monitor readings that indicate the desired comparable change has occurred in the body function being measured.

Trained therapists suggest mental or physical exercises designed to help patients gain more control over their bodies. Patients observe monitoring equipment, which provides feedback about physiological change and helps the individual alter heart rate, skin temperature, or some other targeted state. This process is repeated as often as necessary to effect the desired result, such as reducing pain or modifying other uncomfortable symptoms. The patient learns to connect alterations in thought, breathing, posture, and muscle tension with the desired results. It becomes a case of the mind controlling the body in ways that Westerners thought were impossible only a few decades ago.

What Practitioners Say It Does

Biofeedback therapies were developed to treat a wide range of symptoms and problems, including stress, urinary incontinence, sleep disorders, Raynaud's disease, migraine headaches, hypertension, addictions, vascular disorders, and many others. The therapeutic procedure involves focusing the mind on a biological function and mentally visualizing or picturing the desired change. This might be warming the temperature of one's hands, tightening blood vessels to eliminate headaches, or inducing other physiological events to help relieve the particular disorder.

According to practitioners, biofeedback creates among patients a greater awareness of specific body parts and their functions. With training, increased awareness of physiological functions enables the patient to regulate these functions.

Biofeedback provides a logical approach to resolving many medical problems. When patients are properly trained, they can relieve or eliminate symptoms, replace feelings of helplessness with a sense of renewed control over health, and reduce their own health-care costs.

Research Evidence to Date

It is clear that the use of monitoring devices to provide feedback about internal events is beneficial for many people. There is strong evidence that biofeedback is effective in treating alcoholism, drug abuse, and anxiety. It can lower the physical tension associated with many illnesses and help control high blood pressure and chronic pain.

Well-controlled studies report positive effects of biofeedback in treating Raynaud's disease. Biofeedback can also help people overcome urinary incontinence by developing more effective control of their bladder muscles. It can assist the retraining of body muscles after an accident or surgery, and help train new muscles to take over the function of those that are irreparably damaged.

Researchers say that at least half of those who use biofeedback to treat headaches realize 50 to 80 percent improvement. It should be noted, however, that approximately the same proportion of patients show improvement when treated by relaxation without feedback. Biofeedback is useful also to prevent and reduce migraine headaches in some people. There are still questions about the effectiveness of hand warming as a primary biofeedback therapy for migraine headaches, as clinicians cannot predict accurately who will benefit and who will not.

What It Can Do for You

A primary objective of biofeedback is to promote relaxation with a high level of effectiveness. Although an individual may feel relaxed, biofeedback measuring devices may show otherwise. Because of its ability to measure and report functions of the autonomic nervous system, it may be a more helpful system for many people than is yoga, Zen Buddhism, or simple meditation. It is a no-risk, noninvasive procedure that is worth a try for the problems noted here.

Where to Get It

Most biofeedback therapists are trained as psychologists. The Biofeedback Certification Institute of America recognizes therapists who are properly trained in the technique.

Physicians may know of qualified biofeedback therapists. Also, many psychologists are listed in the Yellow Pages of the telephone directory, and their advertisements may list biofeedback as an available treatment.

Find a biofeedback expert who seems best prepared to meet your individual needs, and with whom you feel comfortable. Look for someone who has had success in treating patients with disorders or health problems similar to yours. Ask questions about the process. A good therapist will willingly describe the procedure, its benefits, and any potential weaknesses without hesitation.

Directories of biofeedback practitioners are available from the Biofeedback Certification Institute of America and the Association for Applied Psychophysiology and Biofeedback:

+ Biofeedback Certification Institute of America (BCIA)
  10200 West 44th Avenue, Suite 304
  Wheatridge, CO 80033
  Telephone: (303) 420-2902
+ Association for Applied Psychotherapy and Biofeedback
  (same address as BCIA)
  Telephone: (303) 422-8436
+ Mind-body Medical Institute
  Division of Behavioral Medicine
  New England Deaconess Hospital
  183 Pilgrim Road
  Boston, MA 02213
  Telephone: (617) 732-9330

15 ⤳
Hypnosis

Like other alternative therapies, hypnosis has existed in one form or another since early recorded history, and like early alternative therapies it was often tied to magic and religion. Hypnosis was an important component of Native American healing rites, when hypnotic states typically were induced through chanting, sometimes in conjunction with hallucinogenic drugs.

Modern medical hypnosis originated with the Viennese physician Franz Mesmer. Mesmer believed that the human body contained "animal magnetism," and that imbalances in magnetic forces were the cause of illness. The therapy he applied, termed mesmerism, involved the use of tranquil gestures and soothing words to relax the patient and to restore balance in the patient's magnetic forces. Although mesmerism did not find long-lasting support, the idea of using a state of altered awareness in medical treatment gradually gained wider acceptance.

What It Is

Hypnosis is a state of focused attention or altered consciousness, a restful alertness in which distractions are blocked, allowing a person to concentrate intently on a particular subject, memory, sensation, or problem. Hypnosis may be used in lieu of anesthetic agents during surgical and dental procedures, often when allergy or some other circumstance prohibits anesthesia. It is also used to reduce stress, pain, and anxiety and to assist in removing undesired habits such as bed-wetting in children or smoking.

Hypnosis is not considered a medical procedure in and of itself. It cannot cure disease and should not be relied on to do so. Rather, it is most widely regarded as a treatment used in conjunction with conventional medicine, and in this capacity it is finding growing acceptance and application.

What Practitioners Say It Does

At the very least, proponents say, hypnosis brings about a state of increased relaxation. Claims about its

Who Can Be Hypnotized?

Roughly 90 percent of the general population can be hypnotized to some degree. Success depends on one's willingness and receptivity to the idea of hypnosis. Children appear to be more easily hypnotizable than adults, primarily because using the imagination comes easily and naturally for them, and because they tend to be creative and trusting.

The Alternative Medicine Handbook

efficacy expand from there. It can serve some as a remedy for addiction, including drug, alcohol, and tobacco dependency. It helps some people maintain diets, relieve stress, and reduce anxiety. It can effectively relieve or eliminate chronic migraines, arthritis, and even warts, which appear to respond to various types of mental suggestion.

There are documented instances of hypnosis analgesia used successfully under varying circumstances. A fifteen-year-old girl who was allergic to pharmacologic anesthesia, for example, completed successful heart surgery with hypnosis as the only analgesic. It enabled her to remain conscious during the four-hour procedure, without so much as an aspirin required during or after the surgery.

Those who study hypnosis explain that it has measurable physiological effects. Beyond its analgesic functions, hypnotic suggestion is known to steady the heartbeat and blood pressure, relax muscles, and reduce bleeding during surgery. Those who have used hypnosis in this capacity report less postoperative pain and faster recovery times than patients using pharmacologic anesthesia.

Proponents of the use of hypnosis during surgery contend that its pain-relieving effects linger indefinitely after emergence from the hypnotic trance. Consequently, they argue, hypnosis should be appropriate and effective in controlling the persistent pain often associated with chronic illnesses such as cancer and arthritis.

Not everyone can be hypnotized. For those who can, however, hypnosis has important benefits. To achieve pain control, for example, hypnosis can be self-induced by patients whenever they feel the need for pain relief. This can help them avoid narcotic dependency and the long-term expense and physical complications of narcotic medication.

Beliefs on Which It Is Based

A frequently voiced concern about hypnosis is that it involves the surrender of control, leaving the subject susceptible to the suggestion of the hypnotist. Precisely the contrary is correct, practitioners say. Control by the subject is the most fundamental underlying precept of

Control

In hypnosis, it is the subject, not the practitioner, who retains control.

hypnosis. The goal of hypnosis is for the subject to *gain* control—over behavior, emotions, or physiological processes. In fact, in medical hypnotic therapy, the patient must master self-hypnosis to employ the technique whenever needed. Effective hypnosis is a therapeutic regimen administered by the individual as well as the medical practitioner.

The self-control behind hypnosis helps people relax and become receptive to suggestion. The suggestion, geared to effect the desired results, may come from the patient or the practitioner. By placing themselves into a deep state of relaxation and focused attention, people learn to control pain or bodily functions, or to diminish situation-specific anxieties, such as fear of flying. People who are afraid to fly can hypnotize themselves and reevaluate their perceptions and attitudes about being in an airplane. They could see the plane as an extension of themselves rather than as a container of fear.

Smokers and overeaters may use hypnotic concentration to adopt healthier attitudes. Hypnotic suggestions might involve seeing the quitting of smoking or overeating as a favor or gift to the body, rather than as a deprivation of its pleasure. By quieting the conscious mind, the unconscious is more open to suggestion. The power of hypnosis is further evidenced by the fact that young hemophiliacs learn to use hypnosis to control their bleeding.

Research Evidence to Date

Because hypnosis has been used for several centuries, it has endured times of ridicule and times of acceptance. The pendulum currently seems to be swinging toward broader acceptance, primarily because solid research now documents the effectiveness and utility of hypnosis for both children and adults. An example of such studies is Stanford University's demonstration of electrical response brain waves. Hypnotized subjects were able to suppress the brain's electrical response to a visual cue by imagining that their view of the stimulus was blocked. This kind of response had been assumed to be involuntary. Hypnotized subjects in the study also were able to control their skin temperature and blood flow.

Studies of the effectiveness of hypnosis in curbing

The Alternative Medicine Handbook

habits such as smoking found a success rate comparable to that of other smoking cessation techniques. One in four people using hypnosis continued to refrain from smoking six months later. Other investigations exhibited similar results, including a 1981 project conducted by Stanford and Columbia Universities involving airplane phobias. Of the 178 subjects who participated in a single-session self-hypnosis training program for aerophobics, more than half remained cured or improved seven years later.

Medical and dental literature supports the efficacy of hypnosis for relief of pain from migraines, dental procedures, labor and delivery, and even surgery. A specialist in family medicine at Case Western Reserve School of Medicine reviewed eighteen clinical trials, finding that hypnotherapy was effective for a wide variety of surgical procedures. The use of hypnotherapy to create the illusion of spinal anesthesia in place of conventional spinal anesthesia was developed by a dentist and psychologist in New York State. A study reported in the *Journal of the American Medical Association* in 1996 showed that hypnosis effectively relieves cancer pain.

Research conducted at Stanford University evaluated the value of hypnosis in reducing pain in children receiving treatments for leukemia. Bone marrow aspiration is a procedure during which, following a local injection of an anesthetic, a large needle is inserted through the skin and into the center of the bone. Usually the hip bone is used. An attached syringe withdraws marrow from the bone for microscopic analysis. Investigators found that hypnosis decreased the children's pain during the procedure by up to 30 percent.

What It Can Do for You

Hypnosis is not a cure-all for physical, emotional, or addictive disorders. It cannot reprogram the body and mind to stop smoking or drinking, for example. It cannot cure serious disease and should never be used as an alternative to conventional medicine. It is not recommended for the treatment of psychosis, organic psychiatric conditions, or antisocial behavior.

It does, however, have significant and meaningful documented benefits. Hypnosis usually produces a state of profound relaxation. Proper hypnotic instruction can refocus attention away from adverse stimuli, including pain, and increase the unconscious mind's receptivity to suggestion. In turn, this can bring about physiological changes such as decreased pulse rate, temperature reduction or increase, and reduced blood flow to specified areas of the body. Hypnosis also is useful against addiction, anxiety, depression, and phobias.

Where to Get It

Several organizations as well as sites on the World Wide Web provide information about hypnosis:
- The American Institute of Hypnotherapy
  1805 East Garry Avenue, Suite 100
  Santa Ana, CA 92705
  Telephone: (714) 261-6400
- The International Medical and Dental Hypnotherapy Association
  4110 Edgeland, Suite 800
  Royal Oak, MI 48073
  Telephone: (248) 549-5594; (800) 257-5467 outside Michigan
- The American Society of Clinical Hypnosis (will provide a list of practitioners)
  2200 East Devon Avenue, Suite 291
  Des Plaines, IL 60018
  Telephone: (708) 297-3317
- The National Guild of Hypnotists
  P.O. Box 308
  Merrimack, NH 03054
  Telephone: (603) 429-9438
- http://ourworld.compuserve.com/homepages/hypnoweb
  An Internet Web site dedicated solely to hypnosis, operated by the International Hypnotherapy Training Center (IHTC) in the United Kingdom.

Imagery and Visualization Techniques

You are lying on the floor, or reclining on a couch, eyes closed, breathing deeply. A soothing voice begins, "Imagine yourself floating, floating with no effort on a calm sea. You feel the water on your back and legs, the sun on your face and chest. You hear the gentle beating of the waves on the faraway shore."

You have just been through an exercise in imagery, a technique, its advocates claim, that can harness our imagination, memory, and senses, all in the service of promoting relaxation, healing disease, and improving control over life and health.

Imagery, rooted in centuries-old techniques, is predicated on the idea that our minds can influence the unseen processes of our bodies, such as the immune system. As do many other forms of alternative healing, imagery relies on the assumption of direct and powerful links between mind and body, some of which are not fully proven. John Milton, the great English poet, wrote that the human mind "can make a heaven of hell. . . ." It is this power that imagery and visualization seek to tap.

What It Is

Imagery is a therapeutic process in which mental pictures play the central role. Imagination and memory are used to mentally taste, smell, see, and hear the images that you or a guide elect to envision. Imagery has been used for medical purposes since at least the thirteenth century, when Tibetan monks meditated on statues of the Buddha, imagining the Buddha healing illnesses. Some imagery advocates believe that the technique was practiced by the ancient Greeks, Romans, and Babylonians.

Two common imagery exercises are palming and guided imagery. In **palming,** you place your palms over your closed eyes. You imagine your mind's field of vision changing first to a color you associate with stress and tension, such as red, and then to a color that you associate with calm and relaxation. Deep blue is an example of a color that many find calming. Visualization of colors that feel calming are thought to promote relaxation.

John Milton, Paradise Lost, 1667

"The mind is its own place, and in itself Can make a heaven of hell, a hell of heaven."

In another exercise known as **guided imagery**, people visualize a goal they want to achieve and then picture themselves achieving it. Guided imagery is not limited to medicine. Athletes often use it, believing that mentally rehearsing a performance increases the chances of success during actual competition. For example, a baseball player might imagine standing at bat, receiving a pitch, and making a hit. A gymnast might imagine going through a complicated routine of floor exercises, without even setting foot on the mat.

An example of guided imagery used often in medicine is the **Simonton method**. Developed in the early 1970s by radiation oncologist O. Carl Simonton and his wife, Stephanie Matthews-Simonton, the Simonton method involves cancer patients conjuring a series of images that depict the body fighting tumor cells. A common exercise, which probably stems from the popular video game, is picturing the cells of the immune system as Pac-Men gobbling up and destroying cancer cells. It is important to note that the Simontons developed their method as a complementary therapy to be used along with, not instead of, mainstream cancer therapy. Their publications advise patients to continue conventional treatment.

Imagery exercises can be practiced by the individual alone or led by a health professional trained in the techniques. Most imagery sessions with a therapist last from twenty to thirty minutes. In self-guided sessions, people usually follow instructions from a book or audiotape.

What Practitioners Say It Does

Imagery can serve as a relaxation technique similar to other mind-body approaches such as meditation and hypnosis. Unlike the latter two, which usually involve focusing attention on one thing for a period of time, imagery often involves frequent changes in focus.

Advocates claim that imagery has physiological and psychological effects. Imagery's physiological effects are similar to those of other relaxation techniques. It can lower blood pressure, alter brain waves, and decrease heart rate. Imagery is said to provide symptom relief of physical problems such as pain and emotional symptoms such as anxiety. It also may improve the effectiveness of pharmacologic or other therapies, as in the example of the Simonton method.

Martin Rossman, M.D., an imagery expert and director of a center for guided imagery in the San Francisco area, claims that the technique can have powerful effects on body and mind, alleviating symptoms and enabling emotional insight. If conjuring an image of food evokes salivation, other mental images should have analogous effects on physiological events.

In addition to physiological results, imagery can lead to psychological and emotional breakthroughs. There are case studies of patients with physical ailments having no apparent medical cause who were able to substantially reduce their symptoms through a program of psychotherapy and imagery.

Beliefs on Which It Is Based

At the root of imagery is a belief common to all mind-body approaches: the idea that the mind influences the health of the body. Mind-body advocates extend the evidence of mind-body techniques causing physiological changes to what they see as its logical conclusion—that these techniques can contribute to the healing of disease, working as complementary therapies to enhance the effectiveness of mainstream treatments. Mind-body efforts, advocates say, can assist conventional therapies to work in less time, with fewer side effects, and with a better chance of success.

Lacking well-documented mechanisms to explain imagery's effects, advocates speculate that the act of imagining an experience stimulates the same part of the brain as does the actual experience. For example, imagining a song and actually hearing the song both stimulate the same part of the brain. This hypothesis has been confirmed using PET (positron emission tomography) scans of the brain. Practitioners speculate that stimulation of higher brain functions leads to activation of the nervous and endocrine systems, which in turn affect bodily functions such as the immune system.

Research Evidence to Date

The best available research indicates that guided imagery has value as a relaxation technique and is therefore a useful complementary therapy. However, carefully designed, scientifically valid studies provide no evidence that guided imagery can help reduce disease, or even influence the effects or action of conventional treatments in serious diseases such as cancer. The Simonton method, for example, has not been proven to increase survival time in cancer patients. Imagery's full potential and limitations as a healing tool await additional, careful research.

What It Can Do for You

Imagery fits the category and achieves the benefits of many other mind-body interventions. Many people find it relaxing. Some anecdotal evidence suggests that it may be able to do more than make people feel good, but scientific research has yet to validate imagery as a healing tool.

Where to Get It

Many therapists are trained to administer imagery techniques, and most explain appropriately that imagery does not cure illness. Rather, it should be used as an adjunct or complement to conventional therapy. When seeking a therapist in your area, it may be helpful to obtain references from past patients. As when engaging any professional, question the therapist about experience, areas of specialization, and professional credentials.

Imagery is inexpensive, particularly if self-taught or self-administered. It is not difficult to learn, and it is safe. The many books devoted to the use of imagery include:

+ Martin Rossman's *Healing Yourself: A Step-by-Step Program for Better Health through Imagery* (Walker, New York, 1987).
+ Michael Samuels' *Healing with the Mind's Eye* (Random House, New York, 1992).

Many audiotapes and videotapes devoted to imagery are available in libraries and bookstores.

Kirlian photography is a dubious technique used to diagnose illness and abnormalities by reading or interpreting "auras" on an exposed photographic plate. Such exposures are created on sheet film placed atop a metal plate when a body part (such as a hand, foot, or fingertip) is pressed against the film. An aura is created around that body part and captured on the film when a high voltage electric current is passed through the metal plate.

Auras created by Kirlian photography are luminous radiations that outline the body part under study. Auras look like multicolored concentric rings, often dominated by blue and white and permeated by dots of other hues.

Many alternative practitioners believe in a variety of life forces, and some extend this concept to the belief that people radiate luminous energy fields. These fields, they say, can be analyzed to provide insight into mental, physical, and emotional states. It is this force that Kirlian photography practitioners believe is captured by the "electronic photography" process. They also believe that images created by this process can be used as diagnostic tools.

What It Is

Kirlian photography first emerged as the result of research conducted by the Soviet husband-and-wife team Semyon and Valentina Kirlian in the late 1950s. Kirlian photography produces images that could be described as being similar to the sun in total eclipse—a dark center where the foot, hand, or finger touches the film, completely surrounded by an "aurora borealis" of color, often showing bright white slivers of light shooting out into concentric circles of increasingly darker shades of blue. Sometimes varying shapes of red, yellow, and white dots of light are seen in the aura. Auras are defined as portraits of the body's bioenergy or life force.

It is these varying images that practitioners in Kirlian photography use to make diagnoses of the patient's biological state, including evidence of disease. Some say that the auras also reflect the person's emotional state and psychic relationships.

What Practitioners Say It Does

Chief among claims for Kirlian photography is that it is a useful means of making medical diagnoses. Promoters contend that mood, energy level, and health can be determined by the color of one's auras. Certain patterns also may signify whether something is wrong inside the body. As proof of this phenomenon, practitioners state that patients with the same illness have similar auras. Conditions identifiable through Kirlian photographs span the medical spectrum. Nutritional deficiencies, mental illness, substance abuse, organ weakness, cancer, and other disorders are all said to show their presence in energy fields. Even states of mind such as confusion and anxiety are claimed to be apparent in Kirlian photographs.

Beliefs on Which It Is Based

The concept that underlies Kirlian photography is the belief that all objects and humans emit invisible auras, thought to define life forces, that can be "captured" and "read." Reading or interpreting the auras provides information about states and characteristics of that object or person.

Research Evidence to Date

Despite the beliefs and efforts of advocates, few members of the traditional scientific community accept the legitimacy of Kirlian photography. Most explain the colorful halos in terms of nothing more than physiological variations on the skin's surface at the time of the photograph. Factors such as moisture, temperature, and pressure, as well as variations in voltage and exposure time, cause color and pattern differences among patients, experts explain.

Rumanian researchers in 1978 claimed that they could detect differences in Kirlian photographs between cancerous and nonmalignant tumors, and said they could detect breast cancer using Kirlian photography with complete accuracy. This approach is claimed by some proponents also to diagnose asthma. Individuals with asthma, they contend, have auras with a recognizable wispy pattern. Claims of the diagnostic value of auras are not taken seriously by scientists.

What It Can Do for You

The general consensus seems to be that, aside from producing a colorful picture of your hand, there is very little that Kirlian photography can accomplish. The process should not be used to substitute for mainstream diagnostic techniques or to determine medical conditions of any kind. Kirlian photography is not a rational option to be considered in place of conventional treatment. Most diagnoses attempted by Kirlian photography can be more easily determined by asking the individual what his or her problem is or by observation. Standard diagnostic procedures such as X rays and blood tests are needed to diagnose serious medical conditions.

Where to Get It

Although not pervasive, there are still some who practice Kirlian photography. They are often found at health fairs. Be wary of Kirlian practitioners who claim to diagnose nutritional deficiencies and then sell expensive supplements.

18 ⤻
Meditation

Although meditation is among the most accepted alternative therapies in mainstream medicine, its origins lie in magic and religion. Shamans, or early priests, meditated while enlisting guidance from the spiritual realm. Every major religion in the world, including Christianity and Judaism, has regarded and utilized meditation as a link to spiritual enlightenment.

Meditation gained serious attention in Western cultures in the 1960s. As word spread of Eastern masters able to perform remarkable feats of bodily control and achieve altered states of consciousness, people in Western countries became increasingly fascinated by meditation. Health practitioners and researchers became interested in understanding how the mind could evoke physiological changes in the body. Meditation's purported ability to achieve physical benefits was a natural springboard for the curiosity and research activity that continues to this day.

What It Is

Meditation has been described in varying, often extreme terms. Viewed by some as a means of maintaining attention pleasantly anchored in the current moment, it has also been canonized as a catalyst for world peace. As emphasized in most Asian traditions, mental control is the foundation of meditation, and mental control also lies behind meditation's application as a complementary healing technique. Mental mastery is believed capable of producing physiological and emotional change. The goal is to improve health in general and facilitate the healing of certain disorders.

Across its many varieties, meditation includes certain common procedures. The meditator sits or rests quietly, usually with eyes closed, in a peaceful environment devoid of distractions. Mental exercises geared to channel concentration and relax the body are performed. The aim is to stay relaxed yet alert. Typically, a focal point of concentration is selected. This can be an object, a word, or a sound, a mantra or action, or merely the rhythm of one's own breathing. Many practitioners also adopt a passive, receptive attitude in which fleeting thoughts are disregarded without reflection. Saint Francis of Assisi likened these thoughts to birds flying overhead that should be observed without "letting them nest in the hair."

What Practitioners Say It Does

Meditation is lauded often as a means of managing stress. Stress is now widely acknowledged as contributing to and exacerbating many health problems (see the introduction to Part III). Therefore, therapies such as meditation have many proponents, because these approaches provide effective relaxation techniques that help patients deal with stressful situations.

During meditation, people learn to redirect their attention to the present, reacting neither to memories of the past nor thoughts of the future. Preoccupation with past and future is believed to be a major source of chronic stress. The mental training that meditation provides teaches individuals to be aware of what causes their stress, thereby giving them a sense of control. Control makes the difference between positive and detrimental stress.

The benefits of relaxation and stress reduction, in turn, appear to reduce levels of stress hormones, improve immune functioning, diminish chronic pain, improve mood, and even enhance fertility. Quieting the conscious mind is believed also to allow the body's inner wisdom, or "internal physician," to be heard. That is, meditation promotes the body's ability to heal itself.

Further benefits attributed to meditation include enhanced immune functioning in individuals with chronic diseases such as cancer and AIDS. Practitioners also claim success with meditation included as part of the treatment of patients with hypertension and heart disease. It is also considered useful in assisting rehabilitative therapies for alcohol, drug, and other addictions.

Devotees say that, with regular, long-term meditation, they experience personal and spiritual growth. They claim richer sensory experiences, greater alertness, and increased mental efficiency, as well as the ability to access deeper levels of awareness. Some even attest to a mystical sense of oneness with God or the universe.

Value of Meditation

Meditation is believed to promote the body's self-healing mechanisms.

Beliefs on Which It Is Based

The major foundation for meditation's popularity, especially as a benefit to personal health, is the belief that the mind can cause changes in the body. Many cultures, particularly those in Asia where meditative strategies have long been included in health regimens, have relied on this idea for centuries. A more recent underlying belief is the idea that stress induces harmful effects on the body. Because meditation emphasizes mental training and relaxation and imparts a sense of control, it is considered a potent agent against stress and anxiety, and therefore has gained widespread acceptance as a valid medical therapy.

Research Evidence to Date

Many studies have documented the correlation between meditation and the reduction of stress, anxiety, and panic states. Research has documented the **relaxation response** produced by meditation and prayer, a response involving decreased heart and respiration rates and eased muscle tension.

Meditation has been shown also to help control negative thinking and assist people in managing potentially stressful situations in a calm fashion.

Research such as that conducted at the University of Massachusetts' Stress Reduction Clinic has produced evidence that meditation helps decrease chronic pain. Meditation performed regularly over an eight-week period reduced participants' pain by as much as 50 percent.

Transcendental Meditation

Amidst meditation's 1960s rise in popularity in the West, a version called transcendental meditation (TM) was founded by Maharishi Mahesh Yogi, a physics scholar from India. TM, based on ancient Indian practice, is similar to other forms of meditation such as Zen, yoga, progressive relaxation, and other means of eliciting deep relaxation.

Meditation is a vital component of TM activity. Its promotional materials claim that TM teaches mastery of the forces of nature, enabling students to become invisible, walk through walls, fly unassisted, and develop "the strength of an elephant." Devotees claim that TM is the vehicle for enlightenment and even world peace.

Accepting these beliefs is not prerequisite to benefiting from the practice of TM. TM's physiological benefits, although not unique to this particular type of meditation, are well documented.

The Alternative Medicine Handbook

Frequent meditation may reduce anxiety, depression, and pain among patients with cancer as well. A 1996 study reported in a journal published by the American Heart Association found that Transcendental Meditation (TM), which involves achieving deep physiological relaxation while remaining alert, reduced hypertension in African-American patients. TM reduced blood pressure better than did progressive muscle relaxation or instruction about healthy living habits.

What It Can Do for You

The relaxation and stress-reduction benefits of meditation are well documented. It has been found to reduce lactic acid levels (high levels of which are associated with anxiety). Mainstream medical practitioners often recommend meditation as an adjunct to conventional treatment or as a preventive health measure. Meditation can ease muscle tension, lower oxygen consumption and heart rate, and with practice decrease blood pressure.

Meditation is often recommended for patients with hypertension or heart disease in conjunction with dietary and other positive lifestyle changes. Regular practice of meditation can enhance one's sense of control and improve self-esteem, thereby serving to empower. Meditation can also engender spiritual calm and growth.

Where to Get It

Assistance with meditation is available from practitioners, including psychiatrists and other mental health professionals, stress-reduction experts, yoga masters, and clinics at many major medical centers and local hospitals. The following organizations offer related services and information:

+ Institute of Noetic Sciences
  P.O. Box 909
  Sausalito, CA 94966
  Telephone: (415) 331-5650
  General resource information about meditation.
+ Institute of Transpersonal Psychology
  P.O. Box 4437
  Stanford, CA 94305
  Telephone: (415) 327-2066

Information about meditation research, activities, and teachers.

✦ Mind-Body Clinic
New Deaconess Hospital
Harvard Medical School
185 Pilgrim Road
Cambridge, MA 02215
Telephone: (617) 632-9530
A medical center treatment program; resource for learning the relaxation response.

✦ Mind/Body Health Sciences, Inc.
393 Dixon Road
Boulder, CO 80302
Telephone: (303) 440-8460
Assistance in organizing workshops, speakers, meditation materials including books and tapes.

✦ Stress Reduction Clinic
University of Massachusetts Medical Center
55 Lake Avenue North
Worchester, MA 01655
Telephone: (508) 856-2656

~19
Placebo Effect

In 1955 a classic study analyzing fifteen investigations of 1,000 medical patients was published by Dr. Henry K. Beecher, a prominent physician at Harvard's Massachusetts General Hospital. He reported that the problems of at least one in three patients were relieved by **placebos,** inert substances often called "sugar pills." Beecher noted that placebos were so powerful that they caused not only positive results but also a broad range of negative side effects.

Although Beecher's study was among the first to document the phenomenon of the placebo response—healing that occurs from patients' beliefs or assumptions that a treatment is effective—doctors had known about and used this phenomenon for many decades. Most physicians practicing in the 1800s and first half of the 1900s maintained a jar of "special" (sugar) pills, which they dispensed when having nothing else to offer. There are many stories of patients returning to a previous doctor to complain that the medicine given to them by their new doctor was not as good as the "special" pills administered by the old doctor.

Since Beecher's article, the placebo response has been studied and monitored closely in clinical investigations. Scientists now believe that the placebo effect is at least twice as common as found by Beecher. A medical literature review of close to 7,000 patients who received treatments later found to be worthless, including a surgical procedure for asthma and a stomach-freezing technique for ulcers, was published recently. Forty percent of the patients reported "excellent" improvement, and an additional 30 percent described "good" results. In all, this is twice the percentage of placebo responses uncovered by Beecher, and a good example of results found routinely today.

In addition to documentation throughout the medical literature, several major texts discuss the placebo response. Yale University physician and professor Howard Spiro and Harvard professor Herbert Benson both have new books out on the placebo effect. In addition, *Mind Body Medicine*, edited by D. Coleman and J.

Gurin (Consumer Reports Books, Yonkers, N.Y., 1993) discusses the observation that the placebo response is ubiquitous in medicine, occurring in virtually every disease, symptom, and ailment.

The placebo effect is the mind in action, causing real and measurable physiological reactions to occur. The placebo response is not an alternative or complementary therapy. It is, however, a fascinating and extremely important phenomenon at the heart of mind-body medicine. *Placebo* comes from the Latin meaning "I shall please." In 1785 the word was first applied as a medical term, meaning "a commonplace method or medicine." By 1811 it had come to mean "medicine prescribed to please the patient, used when physicians had nothing more than sugar-pill promises to help the healing process." Often the sugar pills, backed by patients' confidence in both the physician and the medication, did a very good job indeed.

The placebo response relies heavily on the doctor-patient relationship. Expectation explains similar phenomena involving the patient alone, as occurs when one ingests exotic capsules and achieves the promised result but learns later that the pills were inert.

What It Is

The placebo effect is a striking example of mind over body, of mental processes influencing physical events. It shows us that bodily functions that are amenable to suggestion can be manipulated by passive beliefs or willful efforts of thought. In clinical medicine, placebos act primarily to relieve pain and other symptoms. Neither placebos nor any mind-body effort can fix fundamental biological disorders, cause missing limbs to regrow, make mutated genes revert to normal, or heal shattered spinal cords so that paraplegics can walk again.

In modern clinical research, placebos are crucial to the testing of new drugs. Methodologically sound investigations require that a "control group" of randomly selected individuals receive an inert substance instead of the actual drug. In **double-blind studies**, neither the patients nor the doctors know which group has received the placebos. Only at the study's conclusion, when placebo assignments are revealed, does it become clear to scientists whether a larger percentage of patients who received the drug experienced the hoped-for results than did those receiving the placebo.

What Practitioners Say It Does

Sometimes given deliberately (when physicians had no proven medication) and sometimes by chance (when patients participate in research studies), placebos have worked over the centuries to treat the symptoms of many diseases and disorders. Scientists understand that, although placebos are in fact inactive, their use creates a psychologically initiated response that can relieve the body of pain and other distressing symptoms.

Numerous studies have shown that placebos provide relief from pain, including the pain of arthritis, angina pectoris (severe chest pain, usually caused by heart disease), digestive-tract discomfort, chronic back pain, and cancer pain. One explanation for this effect is the possibility that placebos reduce chronic anxiety, which in turn helps to relieve the perception of pain. Placebos also have been shown to play an important role in addiction, helping drug-dependent patients reduce reliance on the abused substance.

Placebos sometimes hinder as well as help. When a negative effect occurs, a placebo effect is called a **nocebo response**. Nocebos also demonstrate the power of the mind to manipulate attitudes and expectations, this time in a negative manner. A controlled study conducted by the British Stomach Cancer Group provided interesting evidence of the nocebo effect. Thirty percent of placebo-treated patients lost their hair, and 56 percent of the same group reported "drug-related" nausea or vomiting.

There are also documented instances of **voodoo death** in some cultures. Voodoo death occurs when a person believes he has been poisoned or hexed. When victims are cursed by a powerful figure in their society, some actually die soon after the event. One explanation of voodoo death holds that the victim's strong beliefs and fears affect the autonomic nervous system that controls heartbeat, causing the heart to fail and death to occur soon thereafter.

Eventually, scientists hope to pinpoint areas of the brain where love, hope, fear, expectation, ambition, and other emotions reside. Someday the interaction of the brain's billions of neurons with the thoughts, hopes, and expectations of the thinking, feeling mind will be better understood.

Beliefs on Which It Is Based

Many physicians believe that placebos can be traced back to the beginning of the doctor-patient relationship, and before that to the relationship between the individual and the priest or shaman. It is thought that placebos change the perception of pain but leave unaltered its underlying cause. The relationship between patient and physician is believed to have a profound psychological effect on the patient, because the trust, strength, optimism, and hope engendered by that relationship can be powerful catalysts for recovery.

The placebo response appears to be more effective when the relationship between physician and patient is close and trusting. This type of relationship is eroding in today's technologically based, managed-care environment. It still exists in alternative and complementary healing, where it is one of the most positive hallmarks and attractions.

Probably most patients bring their anxieties, fears, expectations, and hopes when they enter a doctor's office. Doctors also have their own beliefs, attitudes, expectations, and methods of communicating. Physicians who truly believe in their treatments and relay that optimism to their patients are better equipped to generate a positive placebo response. If enthusiasm is lacking on either side of the physician-patient relationship, a placebo effect is not likely to occur. Because the vast majority of visits to doctors are for transient problems as opposed to major diseases, the placebo response has great opportunity to influence patients' reactions and well-being.

Theories about how placebos may work adopt the idea that placebos change only perception, and that underlying disease remains unaffected. Details of the relationship between mind and body hold the key to the placebo effect. The sciences of psychiatry and neurobiology eventually will reveal these poorly understood mechanisms.

The placebo may also be looked on as a symbol of the physician's power to heal, or as a function of the patient's suggestibility. For the placebo to be a symbol, however, it must by definition be culturally accepted. The placebo works both ways, for it affects the physician as well as the patient. The placebo tells the patient that the physician is in control, and that the physician can help. It has been suggested that the placebo symbolizes a bond between physician and patient. For the patient to know that a learned physician can maintain caring control may serve as a mental catalyst to promote healing or at least to stimulate its beginning.

Research Evidence to Date

The pain of chronic disease has been studied more closely than that of acute disease. Much more investigation is required. The pain of angina pectoris is remarkably responsive to the administration of placebos. At first, drug therapy for angina usually proves effective in 70 to 90 percent of patients. Gradually, the number of people helped by the new drug diminishes by the 30 to 40 percent of the patients who experience "placebo effectiveness." It is of interest to note that "30 to 40 percent" consistently emerges as the average frequency range with which pain is relieved by placebo.

Studies have attempted to describe a so-called placebo personality. To this end, subjects' personality traits, cultural and socioeconomic status, levels of suggestibility, and anxiety have been studied. Gender, age, and intelligence also were investigated. Most research concluded that no particular characteristics or personality type fits people who respond to placebos. Of all characteristics studied, anxiety was most likely to be related to the effectiveness of a placebo. It is likely that patients with high levels of anxiety, who suffer from considerable amounts of stress, are more susceptible to the placebo effect.

What It Can Do for You

The term *placebo* today has acquired something of a stigma. Many view placebos as ineffective, deceitful remedies. Yet many positive results have come from placebos, including abatement of chronic pain and other symptoms of serious illness. The placebo effect is intriguing, as is the fact that the mind can produce a negative, nocebo response to an inactive or nonspecific drug.

Although many people decry the apparent deception involved in giving placebos, the placebo effect is most likely to produce a positive response in circumstances involving the greatest openness. Placebos work best when patients are provided with a clear understanding of their illness, when family and friends are available to provide moral support, and when patients take some control and maintain hope for a positive outcome.

Most ancient cultures developed a concept of cosmic and bodily energy flow as a means of explaining the world, the body's function, and the relationship between humans and the environment. In early China, this energy was viewed as a vital life force called *qi* (pronounced "chee"), believed to flow throughout the body along energy pathways called meridians. Maintaining smooth and balanced flow of energy, or *qi*, is perceived as necessary to health and well-being. Manipulating *qi* to maintain balance and health is known as *qigong,* which literally means "energy work."

Qigong is a vital part of Chinese medicine and the basis of Asian martial arts. Today it is used widely as a gentle technique to calm the mind and improve stamina. *Qigong* exercises involve combinations of concentrated, controlled breathing with simple, repetitive motions.

During the Cultural Revolution of the 1960s, *qigong* was banned in China. Today, however, it is broadly accepted, not only in China but in many parts of the world. When *qigong* is combined with the calculated, more active motions of ancient Chinese martial arts, it becomes *tai chi* (see Chapter 40), the gentle exercise regimen practiced in cities and rural areas throughout China by people of all ages, including the elderly.

What It Is

Qigong is the willful manipulation of the vital life force called *qi.* There are two types of *qigong*: internal and external. **Internal *qigong*** is practiced alone by the individual to promote self-healing and maintain health through strengthening one's own *qi.* Internal *qigong* can be performed with little or no movement, while sitting, standing, walking, or lying down or during quiet meditation. Its physical component may range from controlled breathing to simple repetitive exercises. The crucial activity, however, is intense concentration focused on moving one's *qi* throughout the body.

External *qigong* involves a special skill developed by master therapists said to externalize or emit their own *qi* and influence the health of other people or even the

A Qigong Exercise

The goal of this exercise is to build up life energy (*qi*) with your breath.

Stand or sit quietly with palms upward, fingertips touching, elbows out, and hands two inches above the navel. While inhaling, raise hands up to the chest. Hold your breath for a moment, turn palms down, and exhale as you move your hands back down to a spot a few inches above the navel. Repeat several times. While performing this exercise, visualize *qi* accumulating in the abdominal region, that part of the body is known in traditional Chinese medicine as the seat of energy, the core from which the vital force springs.

This practice is designed not to fight an existing illness, but rather to increase and strengthen *qi* throughout the body. Stronger *qi* is said to reduce the risk of illness and to enhance well-being.

motion of inanimate objects. *Qigong* masters are teachers, but they can also serve as therapists—"energetic healers" who use their own energy to improve a patient's *qi* and thereby strengthen his or her vitality.

Some *qigong* masters are said to perform great feats. With profound effort and concentration, they send powerful *qi* energy from their bodies into the bodies of others, who are then healed of disease. The transfer of *qi* from master to patient does not require touch. In some respects external *qigong* is similar to psychic healing or psychotherapy, except that external *qigong* assumes an actual healing force or energy flow. This force is both invisible and unmeasurable.

What Practitioners Say It Does

According to ancient Chinese principles, *qigong* improves the flow of *qi* in the body, thereby reducing pain, curing disease, and promoting better health. It is believed that *qigong* works by breaking down energy blockages, enhancing energy flow throughout the body. The improved flow of energy stimulates internal organs and blood, lymph, and nerve-impulse circulation, all of which are deemed important to the maintenance and restoration of good health.

Proponents indicate that *qigong* lowers heart rate and blood pressure, and improves relaxation potential. Specific *qigong* exercises aimed at directing the flow of *qi* to certain areas of the body are used to help prevent tension headaches, constipation, and insomnia. Practitioners describe reports of *qigong* curing cancer; reducing farsightedness and nearsightedness; and successfully treating sinus allergies, hemorrhoids, and problems of the prostate (all highly unlikely). Other reports indicate that *qigong* can lessen the pain of arthritis and migraine headaches and alleviate depression, reduce anxiety, and promote sounder sleep (very probable).

Beliefs on Which It Is Based

Qigong's basic premise is that *qi,* a naturally occurring healing force that exists within the body, can be mobilized by certain exercises or movements combined with meditation and controlled breathing. Another fundamental belief is that activated *qi* increases resistance to disease, improves and maintains overall health, and cures illnesses.

Modern proponents theorize that electrical charges, which they say are responsible for maintaining the proper functioning of organs and tissues, flow along acupuncture meridians and can be influenced by proper *qigong* therapies. A related explanation is that *qi* activates electric currents and stimulates bioelectric conductibility in the body. Others suggest that improving the flow of *qi* modifies brain-wave frequency, heart rate, and the functioning of body organs. It is suggested also that *qigong* may improve resistance to disease and infection because it eliminates toxic metabolic by-products.

Research Evidence to Date

Although *qigong* has been studied extensively in China, many studies were not published and others were not conducted according to international scientific standards. Therefore, they are neither readily available in Western medical literature nor accepted by Western science. Often, studies published in Chinese journals are anecdotal reports of one or a few patients, rather than controlled studies with many subjects. Scientists require rigorous evaluations involving large groups of patients before they will accept a regimen as beneficial.

Qigong proponents in the United States claim in their promotional material that patients who practice *qigong* have better results with conventional therapies for hypertension, heart disease, and cancer than those who do not practice *qigong*, but no data exist to substantiate these claims. Other proponents say that the energy transmitted by *qigong* practitioners to patients can be detected. Acceptance of these claims awaits evidence from controlled studies.

What It Can Do for You

With practice, *qigong* can lower stress levels, reduce anxiety, and provide a feeling of increased well-being and peace of mind. *Qigong* improves overall physical fitness, balance, and flexibility. We do not really know exactly how *qigong* works, or even whether *qi* exists. Regardless, *qigong* strengthens the body, the mind, and the spirit and helps many people feel and function better.

Exactly how and what in the mind and body *qigong* helps is largely a matter of speculation. *Qigong* exercises may induce something like a "relaxation response," the physiological activity, first described by Harvard professor Herbert Benson, M.D., that underlies meditation and deep relaxation.

It is important to note that there is no evidence that *qigong* exercises can increase resistance to illness or cure existing disease, nor is there scientific proof that *qigong* masters can heal patients suffering from serious illnesses. Furthermore, the concept of a channeled flow of energy in the body has not been documented. Nonetheless, it has endured over time and across cultures.

Qigong embodies beliefs that help explain the mysteries of illness and health. Although it is not likely that it can cure serious illness, its ancient techniques can help promote relaxation, increase stamina, and bring about a sense of well-being.

Where to Get It

+ *Qigong* may be self-taught through videotapes and print-ed training materials. These are available at local libraries as well as through the organizations listed below.
+ Many YMCAs and community fitness centers offer *qigong* training.
• The Healing Tao Center in Huntington, New York (516 367-2701), holds classes throughout the United States, in Europe, and in other parts of the world.
+ The American Foundation of Traditional Chinese Medicine in San Francisco (415 776-0502) offers classes and referrals.

ALTERNATIVE BIOLOGICAL TREATMENTS

In some respects, biological therapies have one foot in mainstream medicine and the other in the very different world of alternative health care. Like many mainstream therapies and unlike most other alternative and complementary therapies, alternative biological treatments consist of active chemical substances, or drugs. They are invasive, involving the introduction of pharmacologic substances into the body. They can have powerful physiological effects.

Unlike mainstream therapies, however, alternative biological therapies lack scientifically acceptable evidence of safety and efficacy. According to mainstream scientists, these therapies are not credible, and they have the potential to induce serious harm. Also unlike conventional medicine, alternative biological treatments claim to cure some of today's most significant causes of mortality and morbidity, including AIDS, cancer, heart disease, arthritis, mental illness, chronic pain, and Alzheimer's disease. Of course, such promises cannot be fulfilled. Alternative biological therapists rarely compete with mainstream medicine against serious diseases for which conventional cures exist: there are few alternative therapies for curable diseases.

Alternative biological treatments are fundamentally different from the natural, noninvasive, and gentle holistic care that many desire. Because they are typically recommended by proponents for use *instead* of mainstream therapy, biological alternatives differ importantly from complementary techniques, which are used *in conjunction with* mainstream medical care or as routes to well-being by the healthy. Biological alternatives tend to be applied against life-threatening medical illnesses, whereas complementary techniques are used to abate symptoms or enhance quality of life.

The origins of these biological alternatives vary. Some, like bee venom, which was prescribed by Hippocrates, date back to ancient times. Others are relatively recent in origin and are based on the clinical observations of an individual physician. Cell therapy, the injection of live or freeze-dried animal cells into human beings, was developed by a Swiss physician in the early 1930s. The man who sells shark cartilage treatments as food supplements also wrote a best-selling book in 1992 extolling the product's virtues.

Although the mechanisms proposed for alternative biologicals differ across therapies, most are based on explanations of human physiology and disease that are inconsistent with or unsupported by conventional science. Colon therapy, for example, is based on the idea that high-fat, Western diets lead to an accumulation of a thick, gluelike substance in the colon, which in turn produces disease-causing toxins. The belief in disease-causing toxic material in the body is common in alternative medicine. The idea is not supported by mainstream science.

Biological therapies are often promoted for many different illnesses. This is possible because most proponents of biological alternatives believe that a single underlying problem causes all diseases. Proponents of oxygen therapy believe that insufficient supplies of oxygen in body tissues causes the spread of microorganisms, which, in turn, are responsible for causing a wide range of diseases. Thus, restoring the oxygen supply in body tissues with oxygen therapy is said to preclude development of these diseases.

In other cases, proponents of alternative biologicals take a therapy used in conventional medicine and extend it to conditions for which it has not been proven effective. Chelation therapy, for example, is an accepted treatment for lead poisoning, but not for heart disease as promoted by alternative therapists. Moreover, the mechanism of action proposed for chelation therapy by its advocates is inconsistent with current scientific understanding of heart disease.

Advocates of many biological treatments define their goal as stimulating the immune system so that the body will be able to heal itself. Promoters of enzyme therapy, metabolic therapies, and most other treatments developed in recent decades that reflect mainstream scientific emphasis claim their techniques stimulate immune system activity.

Biological alternatives, like conventional pharmaceuticals, have strong effects on the body. Unlike pharmaceuticals, which must be proven safe and effective before they can be marketed, the treatments in this chapter either have not been evaluated or are disproved. In addition, several are associated with documented potential for serious harm.

Anesthetics used in neural therapy, for example, can provoke serious reactions in people allergic to them. Importing cell therapy to the United States was banned in 1985 because it caused infections and allergic reactions in some patients. EDTA, the active ingredient in chelation therapy, can cause serious kidney damage and death in cardiac patients. Biological dentistry, which involves removing tooth fillings because of their alleged toxicity, has been deemed unethical by the American Dental Association. Studies of bee pollen treatment, oxygen therapies, cell therapies, and the alternative cancer treatment Essiac have found these therapies to be ineffective in the treatment of disease.

Because they are promoted as treatments for serious illnesses, biological alternatives pose an additional threat: patients may delay or bypass potentially helpful mainstream treatment, allowing disease to spread and worsen. Anecdotal reports of cures for the major illnesses dot the promotional material of virtually each and every biological alternative, not only those described in this section. If only a fraction of these reports were valid, humankind would be free of major illness. But anecdotal reports are not equivalent to careful investigations and scientific evidence, so each report should be understood as simply one person's alleged story.

In addition to any harm they may bring, directly or indirectly, biological treatments often are complex, time-consuming, and expensive. Some are not widely available and may involve distant travel to a special clinic dedicated to them. Other biological alternatives, such as chelation and cell therapy, can cost thousands of dollars, usually not covered by standard private or government health insurance.

A selection of today's more popular biological alternatives is presented here. Because those who use or contemplate using biological alternatives typically have been diagnosed with a major illness, it is important to understand that these treatments remain unproven or have been disproved. People should learn exactly what the biological alternative of interest can and cannot accomplish, and potential users should consult with a physician about possible complications or side effects.

∽21
Apitherapy

Apitherapy's roots go back to ancient Egypt. Hippocrates, the famous Greek physician to whom the Hippocratic oath is attributed, used bee venom to treat his patients' arthritis and other joint problems. Some famous rulers throughout history received beestings as a medical treatment, including Charlemagne, Ivan the Terrible, and Charles the Great of England. This long history is continued by practitioners of apitherapy today.

Bee and other insect venom is used in **venom immunotherapy**, which is an accepted means of preventing anaphylaxis (a hypersensitivity to foreign substances, such as happens with allergic reactions to certain proteins in insect stings). However, proponents claim unproven applications for apitherapy, including its use to treat chronic pain, rheumatoid arthritis, multiple sclerosis, lower back pain, migraines, and some dermatologic conditions. Bee pollen consumed internally is also claimed to increases one's energy, endurance, and overall performance. Although practitioner and client testimonials praise the worth of bee-product therapies, no studies document the ability of bee products to cure any ailment or to increase endurance or energy.

Bee products are advertised and distributed through many avenues, including magazines, grocery and health-food stores, and over the Internet. The most commonly promoted bee products are royal jelly, propolis, bee pollen, and raw honey. **Royal jelly** is made by the worker bees and then fed to an ordinary female bee along with the workers' secretions. That female bee then becomes the queen. The royal jelly increases her life span from three months to five years, and she develops the ability to produce twice her weight in eggs. The growth and productivity of the queen bee is due to both the large amount of honey ingested plus the enzymes and hormones in the workers' secretions, which the queen bee receives along with the honey.

Propolis is the waxy material collected by bees from the buds of trees and used to fill cracks in their hives. It has no demonstrated health value.

Promoters claim **bee pollen** contains twenty-two nutrients required by the human body, and that it has five to seven times more protein than beef. A typical dosage of 32 grams, in fact, contains about twenty percent protein, or approximately six grams. This is an extremely small amount. These products have little in the way of nutritional value, but the products sold as pollen do contain protein—in the form of insects, their feces and eggs, rodent debris, and other ingredients.

Promoters also say that **raw honey** is an energy building source, with minerals and seven vitamins from the B-complex group. It actually contains crude sugars—fructose and glucose plus a small amount of sucrose. It is similar to table sugar, which contains pure sucrose. Some bee-product distributors sell each of these items individually, but the ingredients also may be combined and sold as a single product.

Advocates of apitherapy apply bee products in various forms. The two most popular, pills and injections, are given depending on the specific illness. Pills are given for a wide variety of problems such as lack of energy, poor eyesight, memory loss, premenstrual syndrome (PMS), hair loss, and migraine headaches. Injections are typically applied to combat joint pain and arthritis.

What It Is

Pollen is gathered from flowers by bees and brought back to their hive. Harvesters of bee pollen place devices in the hives that strip the pollen from the bees. Because bee pollen comes from many different flowers, its nutritional value varies. Advocates note that the composition of pollen varies according to the geographic region it comes from and the time of year. Despite variation, pollen is composed of sugar, protein, fat, water, vitamins, and minerals. These ingredients may sound healthy, but please note that bee pollen also contains (sometimes sterilized) insect feces and eggs, rodent debris, fungi, and bacteria.

Bee venom therapy is promoted as a cure for joint problems, including rheumatoid arthritis. It has been used in Europe to treat these problems for many years. Proponents of bee venom therapy explain that it works by stimulating the body's immune system. It causes

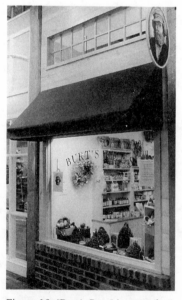

Figure 16 "Burt's Bees" is a retail center for dozens of bee products.

The Alternative Medicine Handbook

inflammation where the venom is injected into the body. In response, the body produces antiinflammatory hormones and other substances to help alleviate the pain and combat the swelling. These hormones are said to be so powerful that they can treat the original condition, such as rheumatoid arthritis. Apitherapy is not a proven form of treatment, nor is it recommended as a therapy for joint diseases or for any other illness.

What Practitioners Say It Does

Supporters of apitherapy claim that it is an effective alternative treatment for many problems and ailments such as arthritis, joint pain, back pain, multiple sclerosis, PMS, and bladder control difficulties. Advocates claim it provides pain relief for arthritis sufferers. Supporters claim that apitherapy is a safe and effective alternative treatment.

Beliefs on Which It Is Based

History has given a great deal of encouragement and support to proponents of apitherapy. Information gathered by supporters has continued to encourage belief in this form of treatment, although the information consists of anecdotal reports rather than scientific research.

Although supporters claim that apitherapy heals and provides relief of symptoms, researchers at major U.S. medical centers as well as a *Consumer Reports* publication have reported allergic and other adverse reactions to bee pollen treatment.

Research Evidence to Date

Studies produced by proponents are criticized by mainstream practitioners because they consist of personal accounts rather than controlled experiments. In contrast, a bee pollen study completed at Louisiana State University involving members of the swim team found no measurable differences in performance between members of the team who used the bee pollen and swimmers who did not. This same study, when repeated with high school swimmers and cross-country runners, produced the same results: no difference in performance was found.

The *Medical Journal of Australia* reported nine

Warning!

Bee product therapies are not harmless. Some people have extreme allergic reactions to beestings that require emergency treatment. Ask your doctor before you try bee-product therapies.

instances of asthmatic attacks and the death of a young asthmatic girl following the use of royal jelly.

What It Can Do for You

Although supporters of apitherapy believe it can increase energy levels, and relieve the symptoms of various illnesses such as arthritis, gout, joint pain, and multiple sclerosis, there is no scientific evidence to support these claims.

Where to Get It

Despite the absence of evidence in support of proponent claims, bee products are widely available. They may be found in pharmacies, in health-food stores, and even in shops that specialize in bee products (Figure 16). For more information regarding proven treatments for rheumatoid arthritis or other joint problems (major ailments for which bee products are recommended), contact your local arthritis foundation. If the White Pages of your telephone book do not contain the listing, call the National Arthritis Foundation (800 933-0032) for the phone number of your local chapter.

For information about treatment for asthma—another ailment for which bee products are promoted—check the White Pages for the American Lung Association.

Biological Cancer Treatments

22

This chapter briefly describes some popular unproven biological therapies used primarily or exclusively against cancer. The other chapters in this section describe additional alternative treatments often applied to treat cancer as well as other illnesses.

These are unproven therapies. People who have been diagnosed with cancer or suspect that they may have cancer should immediately seek qualified care. National Cancer Institute–designated Comprehensive Cancer Centers are within reach of every person in the United States. (Telephone them at 800 4-CANCER, or 800 422-6237, for the center nearest to you.) A visit to confirm diagnoses and treatment plans that can be implemented in your local hospital is important.

Therapies included in this chapter represent a small sample of alternative methods available for cancer. They were selected because they are among those of greatest popular interest today. Laetrile, for example, is not included, because its 1970s popularity waned even before the 1982 publication of a Mayo Clinic investigation showing its ineffectiveness. So-called cancer cures that preceded Laetrile (such as Dr. Ivy's Krebiozen during the 1960s, Hoxsey's Cancer Cure of the 1950s, and Koch's Glyoxylide during the 1940s, among others) also are not included.

Antineoplastons

Stanislaw Burzynski, M.D., Ph.D., emigrated to the United States from Poland in 1970 and became an assistant professor at the Baylor School of Medicine. He isolated a series of peptides (the main component of proteins) that he termed "antineoplastons." He believes that antineoplastons convert cancer cells into normal cells and are deficient in patients with cancer.

Burzynski then developed a cancer treatment aimed at replenishing insufficient antineoplastons. Initially, antineoplastons were isolated from human urine. Later they were synthesized in the laboratory. A main ingredient of antineoplaston therapy is phenylacetate, a fatty acid found in the human body. It is metabolized by the liver and then excreted.

Unproven Biological Cancer Remedies Described in This Chapter

- Antineoplastons
- Cancell
- DMSO
- Essiac
- Hydrazine sulfate
- IAT
- Livingston-Wheeler regimen
- Revici's guided chemotherapy
- 714-X

Burzynski left Baylor to establish his own clinic and research institute in Houston. Both remain open, continually surrounded by controversy. Burzynski and his proponents claim success in curing and bringing about remissions in cancer patients, but others question his credibility as well as his results. Despite laboratory research by a respected scientist who concluded that antineoplastons do not even exist (although peptides are real), despite reports of no apparent benefit by visiting Canadian scientists, and despite a failed National Cancer Institute clinical trial, public interest in antineoplastons remains high.

In 1997, Burzynski was cleared of a seventy-five-count indictment, the latest of several actions brought against him over the years. The recent legal action charged him with violating Food and Drug Administration (FDA) and U.S. Postal Service regulations and judge's orders to stop his selling an unproven therapy. Burzynski's case was no doubt assisted by his large and devoted group of followers. They included desperate patients whose claims of government suppression of this unproven method were well-publicized to Congress and nationally.

Antineoplaston therapy is given only in the Burzynski clinic. Because it remains unproven as well as popular, there is a pressing need for solid research data. Although the FDA granted Burzynski permission to conduct a clinical trial of antineoplastons at his Houston Institute, and despite claims of thousands of cures over the past several years, only recently have patients been placed on the study by the Burzynski clinic.

Therefore, real documentation of patients' medical status before and after antineoplaston therapy does not yet exist. It would not be difficult to replace claims with data, and one must wonder why the Burzynski clinic waited so long to take advantage of this legitimate and easily managed opportunity.

Although there are no hard data to support the merits of antineoplastons as a cancer treatment, the National Cancer Institute is conducting laboratory investigations of these peptides.

Cancell

Cancell, a dark brown liquid, is another well-known biological remedy. It is especially popular in the

Midwest and in parts of Florida. Also called Entelev, Formula JS 114, Jim's Juice, Crocinic Acid, and Sheridan's Formula, Cancell was envisioned in 1936 by James Sheridan, a chemist. The idea came to him in a dream that he said was inspired by God.

Proponents believe that Cancell returns cancer cells to their "primitive state," where the Cancell digests them and renders them inert. However, FDA analyses revealed that Cancell is composed of common chemicals (sulfuric acid, nitric acid, potassium hydroxide, sodium sulfite) and that no basis for its claimed effectiveness against cancer exists. There is no evidence that Cancell works against cancer or any other disease.

DMSO

DMSO (dimethyl sulfoxide) is an industrial solvent, similar to turpentine. A by-product of paper manufacturing, it was first synthesized in 1866. As medication, DMSO was used initially in the early 1960s. Following FDA approval for experimental use, it was applied in topical form to relieve pain, reduce swelling, heal injuries such as muscle strains and sprains, and treat arthritis.

Today, DMSO is approved only to treat interstitial cystitis (a bladder disorder) and as veterinary therapy to reduce swelling in horses and dogs. It is under study for conditions including arthritis, sprains, and a skin disorder known as scleroderma. DMSO is also used to deliver drugs through the skin and to preserve living cells when they are frozen.

DMSO has been proposed as a cancer treatment, although evidence for its efficacy as a cancer treatment is scant to nonexistent. DMSO is considered an unproven and ineffective method of treating cancer.

DMSO can be obtained in health-food stores and other retail and mail-order outlets. In its commonly sold forms, DMSO can have unpleasant side effects, including burning and itching, and it can cause a powerful, garliclike odor in the breath and skin lasting for several days. It may also contain impurities. Probably the most serious potential danger associated with DMSO is that patients may avoid or delay receipt of medical care in a timely fashion.

Essiac

Essiac was first popularized in the early 1920s by Renée Caisse (Essiac is Caisse spelled backwards), a Canadian nurse. Caisse claimed that she received the formula from a woman who used it to cure her own breast cancer. This woman, in turn, is said to have been given the unnamed product by a Native American healer living in Ontario, Canada. Caisse first produced Essiac in the form of a tea. Since her death in 1978, several companies started manufacturing Essiac, and their products still compete, each claiming to be the original formula.

Essiac is comprised of four herbs: Indian rhubarb, slippery elm, sorrel, and burdock. Caisse believed that Essiac worked by attacking the tumor directly, first hardening it, then causing it to soften and break up, and finally discharging it from the body. However, scientific investigation has failed to confirm these claims.

Although the herbs in Essiac have shown some anti-tumor effect in the test tube, this is true of many investigated compounds, the great majority of which are found not to work as anticancer agents in humans. A 1982 study by the Canadian government of cancer patients taking Essiac found that patients did not benefit from it, and laboratory research conducted in 1983 by the U.S. National Cancer Institute found no merit to the product.

Essiac is sold in health-food stores and catalogs as a nutritional supplement. In Canada, it is also available through a program for patients for whom no effective conventional cancer treatment exists. Because it is unproven as a cancer therapy, companies making or selling Essiac may not make claims for its medicinal value. If you plan to try Essiac, inform your physician.

Hydrazine Sulfate

Hydrazine sulfate came to prominence as a cancer therapy around 1970, promoted by Joseph Gold, M.D., a cancer researcher in Syracuse, New York. Hydrazine sulfate is an industrial chemical, used as rocket fuel during World War II. Through a series of studies, Gold developed the idea that hydrazine sulfate could slow the weight loss and wasting away of the body, known as cachexia, that often accompanies advanced stages of cancer. He also believed that hydrazine sulfate could enhance the effectiveness of other drugs.

Working initially with terminally ill patients in the 1970s, Gold and other researchers in the United States and Russia found that hydrazine sulfate appeared to inhibit both cachexia and tumor progression when compared with other methods. However, investigations conducted at the Memorial Sloan-Kettering Cancer Center in New York, also in the early 1970s, found no positive effect for hydrazine sulfate in treating cancer patients.

In 1994 three methodologically sound studies involving a combined total of 636 cancer patients were published. Each of the three found no positive effect for hydrazine sulfate. As of this writing, hydrazine sulfate is considered a disproved and ineffective treatment for cancer.

IAT

Immunoaugmentative Therapy (IAT) was developed by Lawrence Burton, Ph.D., a cancer researcher at St. Vincent's Hospital in New York City. The goal of IAT is to balance four blood protein components in the belief that this balance enables the immune system to fight cancer most effectively. Burton established his own clinic on Long Island and then moved to Freeport, Grand Bahamas, in 1977. He patented the ideas behind IAT and refused to share or discuss them with other cancer researchers, making his claims particularly difficult to evaluate.

IAT consists of a mixture of four components, which are proteins and tumor antibodies derived by centrifuge from the pooled blood of healthy donors. Patients receive daily injections of this compound. Burton claimed that IAT's tumor antibodies fight cancer while its protein removes a "blocking factor" that prevents the patient's immune system from recognizing and fighting cancer cells. Although more than 5,000 patients were said to have been treated in the Bahamian clinic, little documentation exists of Burton's methods or results.

There is no scientific evidence that Burton's methods cure cancer or prolong life in cancer patients. Moreover, an important tenet of his theory, that tumors produce "blocks" that hide cancer cells from the immune system, has been proven false. Scientific research on the immune system and its relationship to cancer continues. His therapy began to decline in popularity in the 1980s as other biological alternative cancer treatments, such as Burzynski's antineoplastons, rose to prominence. Burton died in 1993. Despite this and the absence of evidence that IAT can cure cancer by "augmenting" the immune system, the Burton clinic remains open.

Livingston-Wheeler Regimen

Virginia Livingston-Wheeler trained as a physician in New York City. She came to believe that cancer was caused by a microbe, a living, microscopic organism that lives in patients' blood and body tissues. Although mainstream scientists deny its existence, she claims to have seen this microorganism through a special "dark field" microscope.

For many years prior to her death in 1990, she ran the Livingston-Wheeler clinic in San Diego (since then, others have taken over management of the clinic), treating patients twice a week with a vaccine made from each patient's urine. The injected vaccine was used to attack the bacterium that Livingston-Wheeler believed caused cancer. (However, bacteria do not cause cancer.) Treatment also includes antibiotics and numerous additional items, along with a restricted diet. In a controlled study of end-stage cancer patients, patients on the Livingston-Wheeler regimen lived no longer than, and displayed an inferior quality of life to, similar patients treated conventionally.

Revici's Guided Chemotherapy

The cancer therapy developed by Emanuel Revici, M.D., has been hailed by some as being based on an understanding of chemistry that is sophisticated and ahead of its time, and by others as simply another in a long line of dubious cancer therapies.

Revici, a native Romanian who immigrated to the United States in 1947, practiced medicine in New York until he was close to 100 years of age. His clinic continues to operate under the direction of other physicians who use his methods. Revici first published his theory of cancer in a 1961 book, *Research in Physiopathology as a Basis for Guided Chemotherapy with Special Application to Cancer* (Van Nostrand, Princeton, N.J., 1961).

Revici's theory of tumor origin and treatment is quite complex. According to his own summary of his ideas, tumors are either anabolic or catabolic. In science, anabolic processes turn one substance into another useful substance, while catabolic processes change substances into material that is excreted by the body. In Revici's view, anabolic tumors and processes are marked by an excess of sterols, which are a type of lipid, or fat. Cholesterol is an example of a sterol. Catabolic processes, on the other hand, are marked by an excess of fatty acids, another type of lipid. Revici believed that men and lean people are more likely to have catabolic tumors, while women and heavy individuals have anabolic ones.

The Revici method uses sterols to treat excessive fatty acids, or tumors of catabolic character, and fatty acids to treat excesses of sterols, or cancer of anabolic character. Revici expanded his theory of anabolic and catabolic processes to diseases beyond cancer, including radiation burns, osteoarthritis, and AIDS, among others.

Revici's therapy has been labeled unproven by the American Cancer Society, and it received a negative evaluation in a 1965 article in the *Journal of the American Medical Association*. More recent evaluations have not been conducted. Despite these negative views of Revici's cancer therapy, several mainstream chemists have endorsed Revici's understanding of lipid chemistry and noted that his work anticipated that of other scientists on the properties of fatty acids. Revici's therapy has not been subjected to clinical trials to evaluate its efficacy, and it remains an unproven method of cancer treatment.

714-X

714-X is the name given to an alternative product developed by Gaston Naessens, a French microbiologist now residing in Quebec, Canada. Naessens invented the "somatoscope," a microscope he claimed enables the visualization of otherwise invisible blood particles he called "somatids." He used the somatoscope routinely to determine whether treatment with 714-X, a mixture of nitrogen and camphor (to deliver the nitrogen), was working for each particular patient. Naessens theorized that cancer cells are deficient in nitrogen, and that injecting 714-X into the lymph system would convert them to normal cells. There is no scientific evidence in support of the efficacy of this method.

23

Biological
Dentistry

Biological dentistry is the replacement of dental fillings with nonmetallic material. It stresses the belief that materials currently used in fillings, such as mercury, tin, copper, silver, and sometimes zinc, contain toxins that cause hidden dental infections, which pose serious health risks to the body's organs and physiological systems. Advocates of biological dentistry believe that accepted forms of dental treatment may harm not only the teeth and mouth, but also the health of the entire body. They also believe that physical problems in the body manifest themselves in the mouth.

What It Is

Biological dentistry is the use of alternative treatments for problems of the teeth, gums, jaws, and mouth as well as disorders throughout the body. Biological dentists believe that treating the mouth is a method of treating the body. Some proponents believe that biological dentistry's alternative methods can alleviate symptoms of diseases outside the oral cavity, and sometimes even cure those diseases.

Examples of diseases and problems that biological dentists aim to cure include tinnitus (a ringing noise in the ear), vertigo, epilepsy, hearing loss, eye problems, sinusitis, joint pain, heart disease, kidney problems, and digestive disorders.

In addition to traditional dental care, biological dentists apply several alternative forms of treatment such as neural therapy, oral acupuncture, cold laser surgery, homeopathy, and other unconventional techniques. With these alternative treatments they strive to treat the whole patient's medical as well as dental problems:

Neural Therapy Based on the belief that biological energy flows throughout the body but can become imbalanced or short-circuited, neural therapy is applied to restore that balance. Biological dentists inject a local anesthetic around the tooth thought to correspond to a particular body part or organ in efforts to remove the block and restore energy flow.

Oral Acupuncture This procedure involves the injec-

The Premise

Biological dentists believe that the material used to fill cavities causes cancer, Alzheimer's disease, and almost all other chronic illnesses.

tion of saline water, weakened local anesthetics, or homeopathic remedies into acupoints (acupuncture points) in the mouth (see Chapter 1). Oral acupuncture injections are used to relieve pain during dental procedures and treat sinusitis, allergies, digestive problems, and neuralgia (pain from a damaged nerve).

Cold Laser Surgery This alternative form of acupuncture is much like oral acupuncture, but without the needles (injections). It involves the use of a laser light beam aimed at an acupoint. Proponents claim that cold laser therapy kills bacteria associated with dental work, aids in wound healing, and reduces swelling. It is also applied to treat TMJ (temporomandibular joint syndrome).

Homeopathy Homeopathic remedies (see Chapter 4) are used to relieve pain associated with teeth, gum, jaw, or other mouth problems. It is used only as a temporary remedy until dental treatment can be obtained.

Mouth Balancing This procedure includes analyzing the muscles associated with the mouth and the skull, and creating orthopedic braces for the mouth to realign the jaw and alleviate problems such as TMJ, headaches, eye problems, and over- or underbite. Although aspects of mouth balancing sound similar to methods used in the branch of conventional dentistry called orthodontics, mouth balancing is not included among the various treatments used in mainstream dentistry, as its procedures and especially its goals are not considered acceptable.

Nutrition Biological dentistry includes the use of nutritional supplements such as magnesium, selenium, vitamins C and E, folic acid, and digestive enzymes. These are used to treat the presumed mercury toxicity, which is believed to be caused by traditional cavity fillings. The supplements are thought to assist the excretion of mercury from the body and to encourage healing of presumably damaged tissues throughout the body.

What Practitioners Say It Does

Proponents of biological dentistry believe that conventional dentistry causes most of the dental and medical problems that people experience. They say that alternative biological dentistry can cure these problems.

Beliefs on Which It Is Based

Biological dentistry is based on alternative beliefs concerning the cause of disease. Problems treated by biological dentists and their understanding of what causes these problems are given below.

Infections Lie under the Teeth Proponents believe that bacteria remaining from previous dental procedures, or new bacteria, may result from conventional materials used in root canal work or to fill cavities. Toxins are thought to leak from the conventional filling material and harm the immune system, weakening the body and increasing its susceptibility to disease.

Each Tooth Relates to a Particular Body Organ In the 1950s a German doctor who advocated biological dentistry theorized that each tooth in the mouth relates to a specific acupuncture meridian, much in the way that acupoints are believed related to distant body parts. Therefore, he conjectured, an infected tooth means that the corresponding organ also is infected. He proposed that treating the infected tooth would simultaneously treat its corresponding diseased organ.

Root-canal Procedures Cause Illness All root canals are said to cause infections. Resulting leakages of toxins throughout the body are believed to cause illnesses such as diseases of the nervous system, heart, kidney, uterus, or endocrine system.

Dental Replacement Materials Are Toxic It is believed that dental amalgam fillings may release mercury, tin, copper, silver, and sometimes zinc into the body (see Chapter 8 on dietary supplements for a review of the body's need for these minerals), and that these materials can corrode, break up into potentially harmful, charged atoms, and travel into the central nervous system. Once there, proponents believe, charged atoms inhibit the body's ability to function normally.

Dental Replacement Materials Are Not Biologically Compatible Filling a cavity can cause headaches and allergic reactions such as food allergies and sinusitis. Biological dentists recommend replacing metal fillings with "natural, nontoxic, biocompatible" material.

Electricity Is Created by Dental Fillings (electrogalvanism) Proponents claim that saliva and replacement materials can interact to become electrically conductive and, in essence, form a battery. This biological battery, it is believed, may cause lack of concentration, memory loss, insomnia, psychological problems, tinnitus, vertigo, epilepsy, hearing loss, and eye disorders.

Temporomandibular Joint Syndrome (TMJ) Misalignment of the teeth, jaws, or muscles may be caused by poor dental work, tooth decay, or growth problems of the jaw. Realignment techniques include cold laser treatment and craniosacral therapy (see Chapter 35).

Research Evidence to Date

Proponents believe that materials used in traditional dentistry may cause most degenerative diseases, including cancer and Alzheimer's disease. Dentist and patient testimonials to this effect are presented by advocates because no scientific data support their claims. Scientific research has disproved the claims of biological dentistry. In 1987, the American Dental Association (ADA) amended its code, declaring the removal of clinically serviceable mercury amalgams to be unethical. Dentists who remove serviceable fillings may have their licenses rescinded.

Several scientific studies have shown, contrary to the claims of biological dentistry, that dental amalgam is well accepted physiologically and does not hinder wound healing following dental work. Moreover, the National Institutes of Health (NIH) held a conference in 1991 on "The Effects and Side Effects of Dental Restorative Materials." These national experts, following study and discussion, concluded that there is no evidence to support the idea that dental fillings cause problems.

What It Can Do for You

Advocates claim that biological dentistry is a healthier alternative to conventional dentistry. Having one's dental fillings removed and replaced may cause pain in the mouth as well as the pocketbook, but research shows that it helps neither dental nor medical problems.

It is important to note that toxicity is a function of amount. Tiny fractions of many minerals are required by the body, but ingesting large amounts of those same minerals can be poisonous (see Chapter 8). The amount of minerals released by dental fillings, if any, is too small to have any impact on body function.

Where to Get It

For information about modern dentistry, contact the American Dental Association (800 621-8099).

A copy of the NIH report "Effects and Side Effects of Dental Restorative Materials," *National Library of Medicine Bulletin* (1991), may be obtained from the National Library of Medicine, 9000 Rockville Pike, Bethesda, MD 20892.

24 ⌒

Cell Therapy

Sometimes called live cell therapy, cellular therapy, or fresh cell therapy, cell therapy is not approved for use in the United States. This practice of injecting live or freeze-dried cells from animals' healthy organs, fetuses, or embryos to promote healing and youthfulness in humans is used extensively in Europe. It was banned in the United States in 1985 because it lacked proven benefit and caused serious infections and allergic reactions.

What It Is

In 1931 the Swiss physician Paul Niehans developed cell therapy during a medical crisis to help a patient with damaged parathyroid glands. He injected a saline solution containing ground-up parathyroid cells from a steer calf. Niehans attributed the patient's recovery to the parathyroid cell injection.

Niehans was motivated by that success to apply cell therapy to other problems. He developed an extensive cell therapy program to treat degenerative diseases and promote youthfulness generally. Therapy consisted of injections of cells taken from fetal lambs still in the womb of freshly killed mother sheep. Niehans's therapy, delivered in his costly Swiss spa, achieved great popularity and attracted the famous and wealthy. Several world leaders were treated there, including President Dwight D. Eisenhower.

Because the useful life of animal cells for transplantation is extremely short, and because cell rejection may occur in the recipient and can create problems, a method to freeze-dry cells was developed in 1949. This procedure reduced but did not eliminate side effects such as the **immune rejection reaction**, a problem associated with all types of organ transplants and cell therapies. Later, a different type of cell therapy was developed. It employs animal cell extracts in conjunction with animal antibodies, and proponents say it is free of side effects.

Some practitioners today rely on live animal cells harvested from specific organs of sheep or pigs to treat human patients. Others prefer freeze-dried cells, which

The Alternative Medicine Handbook

sometimes are filtered to remove components most likely to create immune rejection reactions.

What Practitioners Say It Does

Proponents claim that injected animal cells can stimulate the immune system, which protects against disease and enhances overall health. They further believe that, through improved health brought about by cell therapy, patients with serious illnesses such as cancer may be better able to face the rigors of traditional cancer-fighting treatment.

Cells injected into the body are believed to seek out the targeted weak or damaged organ and stimulate a healing process. The cells of a particular animal organ are believed to enter that organ in the patient, helping it to recover or thrive. Injected animal kidney cells, for example, are said to migrate to the human kidney, and animal liver cells to the human liver. Niehans believed that the women he treated for menopausal difficulties rarely developed any type of cancer. He attributed this phenomenon to the benefit of injected ovarian cells taken from sheep.

Cell therapy proponents claim that the repair of damaged organs usually is accomplished with less than half a dozen injections. Therapy designed to promote general youthfulness requires at least six months and may continue for as long as two years. Injections are said to retard aging by stimulating and helping certain body tissues retain fluids.

Some proponents believe that cell therapy increases vitality, stamina, skin tone, blood supply, and a general sense of well-being. Enhanced sexual function and reversal of male impotence also have been claimed. Many other successes in treating various diseases are noted, ranging from cancer to Down's syndrome. Finally, as is true of almost all alternative therapies, some proponents speak of cell therapy's value in treating AIDS.

Beliefs on Which It Is Based

Even proponents of cell therapy are not certain why or how the therapy might work. A few theories are suggested, among them that it enhances the immune system, targets organ-to-organ healing, and restores youth and vitality by donating young cells.

If diseases such as cancer result from immunologic deficiencies, proponents conjecture, cell injections from cancer-resistant animals might help increase human resistance to disease. That was the logic behind Niehans's early efforts to develop cell therapy, and present-day practitioners continue to believe that cell therapy stimulates the immune system, thus preventing disease and improving overall health and quality of life. Furthermore, proponents say that RNA (nucleic acids that help control chemical activities in cells) from healthy cells injected into cancerous tissues reduces malignancy.

Cell therapy advocates believe that animal organ cells migrate to comparable human organs. Thus, they claim that specific organ cell therapy can strengthen the recipient organ and promote organ healing and regeneration.

Research Evidence to Date

Claims about cell therapy are based primarily on anecdotal reports, with success stories publicized by physicians in Mexico, the Bahamas, England, and Germany. Niehans claimed that he successfully treated 30,000 patients, but no research supports that contention. The famed South African heart surgeon, Christiaan Barnard, developed a special interest in cell therapy, and in 1988 promised that the following year would bring corroborating research evidence of cell therapy's viability. To date, no such research has been reported.

One study that did appear in a scientific publication, the journal *Pediatrics*, tested the long-claimed benefits of cell therapy in children with Down's syndrome. Children who received cell therapy were compared with those who did not. Unfortunately, no improvement in IQ; motor, language, or social skills; memory; or growth was found for children receiving cell therapy.

What It Can Do for You

The basic value of cell therapy, according to proponents, is its ability to help ward off or fight disease, restore damaged organs, and promote increased vitality

WARNING!

Cell therapy may have harmful side effects. Some patients have suffered serious infections and allergic reactions.

The Alternative Medicine Handbook

and well-being. After many decades of use, however, the value of cell therapy in curing disease, promoting rejuvenation, or providing any health benefit is yet to be documented.

Where to Get It

Though cell therapy is not legally available in the United States, clinics in Mexico, the Bahamas and Europe do offer it. Before considering its use, you should discuss the subject with a physician whom you know and who knows your medical history. Prior consultation with your financial advisor also is recommended. Cell therapy treatments for "restoration of youth" at European spas cost thousands of dollars for each treatment and have not been proven to retard the effects of aging or to prolong life.

25 ⟩

Chelation Therapy

It is referred to by some practitioners and clients as the human "tune-up." *Chelation* comes from the Greek word "chele" for "claw." When chelation chemicals are introduced into the bloodstream, they bind (claw) to iron in the blood and are later excreted from the system.

Chelation therapy has been a proven treatment for lead and other heavy-metal poisoning for half a century. Injected into the bloodstream, chelation chemicals extract harmful overdoses of minerals, enabling their eventual excretion. Chelation is still used today as an approved treatment for heavy-metal toxicity. The danger of potentially fatal kidney damage from chelation is outweighed in these cases by the even more serious toxicity of the metal poisoning.

Some practitioners, however, claim that chelation can treat illnesses and problems other than metal toxicity. Coronary artery disease is primary among these illnesses. Based on the idea that chelation chemicals may remove harmful plaque from the arteries, it is promoted as an alternative to coronary bypass surgery and angioplasty. Chelation is advertised also as a treatment for thyroid disorders, multiple sclerosis, muscular dystrophy, high cholesterol, psoriasis, hypercalcemia, hardening of the arteries, cancer, Alzheimer's disease, and many other disorders. The rationale for these applications is not clear. Scientific data do not yet support the value of chelation therapy for these problems or for any disorders other than heavy-metal poisoning. This chapter concerns chelation only for these unproven applications.

What It Is

Chelation therapy involves intravenous injection of a solution of ethylene diamine tetraacetic acid (EDTA), also termed edetic acid, into the bloodstream. The solution may contain other vitamins and supplements at the practitioner's discretion. In the bloodstream, the EDTA is said to attach itself to coronary plaque or other unwanted materials, and then is excreted in the urine within forty-eight hours.

The procedure requires a clinic visit of approximately three hours. Depending on the doctor's recommendation, three or more visits each week may be prescribed. Many patients receive forty or more treatments, with an average total cost of $3,000 to $4,000.

What Practitioners Say It Does

Proponents claim that EDTA, when used to treat hardening of the arteries, extracts calcium from cells in the walls of the arteries, thus reducing arterial blockages. Advocates claim that chelation is a safe, economical, and effective alternative to angioplasty or bypass surgery. Proponents also claim that EDTA is an effective therapy for many other diseases, such as those listed above.

Beliefs on Which It Is Based

In the 1950s, a doctor practicing in Detroit, Michigan, noticed that patients who received chelation therapy for lead poisoning also experienced relief from angina (chest pain due to inadequate oxygen in the heart muscle). From this he theorized that the chelation might remove calcium, thereby reversing the problem and causing the pain to abate. His work and that of others resulted in the belief among some that chelation therapy is a viable alternative for the treatment of heart and circulatory problems. The rationale for the use of EDTA to treat other diseases has not been provided. Practitioners base their claims on reports of their own experience or that of others.

Chelation therapists have reported various positive results in their patients, including relief from angina and arthritis; diminishing of gangrene; improved memory, sight, hearing, and smell; and increased energy. However, negative effects have also been reported by mainstream medicine, the American Heart Association, and physician groups.These include bone marrow damage, kidney failure, irregular heart rhythm, severe inflammation of EDTA intravenous sites, anemia, and death from the procedure.

Research Evidence to Date

The positive results reported by proponents of chelation therapy have been criticized as based on selected, inadequate studies reported in proponent books rather than in the scientific literature. In 1993 a review was conducted of all chelation therapy studies reported during the previous thirty-seven years. It concluded that scientific data did not support claims of chelation as an effective treatment for heart problems. Both a Danish investigation and a 1994 double-blind investigation of chelation therapy in patients with intermittent claudication (a condition in which circulation to the legs is impaired) found no significant differences between EDTA and a placebo (an inert substance with no active ingredient; see Chapter 19).

What It Can Do for You

Research does not yet support chelation therapy as a viable method of treatment for illness other than toxic metal poisoning. It may produce toxic effects, including kidney and bone marrow damage, irregular heart rhythm, severe inflammation of the veins, and even death. Proponents point to serious toxicity associated with major surgical cardiac procedures and to their own success in treating patients with chelation over the years.

It is estimated that tens of thousands of Americans seek chelation treatment for heart disease. These large numbers alone point to the urgent need for further scientific investigation.

Where to Get It

Chelation therapists have a national organization that can provide information:
+ The American College for Advancement in Medicine
  23121 Verdugo Drive, Suite 204
  Laguna Hills, CA 92653

For information about mainstream treatments for heart disease and other illnesses, look in the White Pages of your telephone book for the disease-related organization concerned with your particular ailment. An example is:
+ American Heart Association
  7272 Greenville Avenue
  Dallas, TX 75231
  Telephone: (214) 373-6300 or (800) 242-8721

Colon/ Detoxification Therapies

References to colon therapy appear in historic accounts dating back to ancient Egypt and Greece. For centuries, physicians have administered enemas as internal body baths. Although the technology of colon therapy has changed over time, the basic premise—internal cleansing and purification—remains the same.

Introduced to the United States in the 1890s, colon therapy rapidly gained wide popularity. People, healthy and sick, flocked to health spas to be cleansed and rejuvenated. Colon therapy was used to treat heart disease, high blood pressure, arthritis, depression, and various infections. With the development of antibiotics in the 1940s, colon therapy lost its appeal and faded, albeit temporarily, into the background.

Today, colon therapies are readily available in spas, specialty clinics, and other settings, and colonic irrigation is a fundamental component of naturopathic therapy and a popular treatment for constipation. The procedure is said to detoxify the large intestine and establish a healthier, better functioning colon. Proponents call detoxification an integral part of health maintenance and preventive health care. It is estimated that tens of thousands of people in the United States seek colon therapy.

The American Colon Therapy Association has more than 500 members. Colon therapists are licensed in some states. Reputable clinics state that they use Food and Drug Adminisatration (FDA)-approved equipment and disposable applicators. Appointments are recommended twice yearly, or when changes in one's diet occur.

What It Is

Colon therapy, also called "colonic irrigation," "high colonic," or "detoxification therapy," is the cleansing of the large intestine (colon) by flushing out "built-up waste." This is accomplished with water or herbal solutions usually administered rectally. The colonic practitioner, also called a colonic hygienist or colon therapist, helps the client insert plastic tubes into the rectum. The water is then pumped in by a machine or infused with the help of gravity.

Alternatives

Consumption of particular herbs or other laxative-type substances by mouth is another route to colon cleansing.

Filtered water, sometimes containing herbs, enzymes, or other substances, is sent through one of the tubes until the colon, five feet in length, is full. The therapist then massages the colon through the abdomen. After an allotted amount of time, the water is eliminated through another tube. This procedure is repeated, using more than a total of twenty gallons of water per session. The average session requires forty-five to sixty minutes.

What Practitioners Say It Does

Advocates refer to colonic irrigation as a "detoxification procedure." It is said to loosen and remove accumulated waste from the folds of the colon. Because proponents believe that colon therapy helps detoxify the body, allowing natural healing to occur more efficiently, colon therapy can be applied as a primary form of treatment. It is also used as a complementary therapy, a preventive measure, and as an aspect of hygienic routine.

Beliefs on Which It Is Based

Proponents believe that the typical diet in contemporary America consists of high "mucoid-forming foods" such as meat and other fat-containing products, and that it is too low in fiber. This nutritional imbalance causes matter to remain in the colon. As it accumulates, this matter becomes a thick, gluelike substance that remains stuck inside the colon walls. The buildup of this substance eventually causes a condition that proponents term "autointoxication." Autointoxication is a process in which toxins produced by the gluey substance are absorbed into the bloodstream. Proponents believe that through this route they may poison the body and cause illness.

Research Evidence to Date

There are no data in support of the claims or beliefs on which colon therapy is based. Research, however, does dispute these claims, and mainstream medicine warns against use of this procedure. When the resurgence of colon therapy occurred in the early 1980s, some practitioners failed to maintain sanitary conditions. Illness and death resulted. The *Journal of the American Medical Association* in 1980 reported the deaths of two women as the result of receiving coffee enemas from an alternative clinic. In 1981, the Colorado *Morbidity and Mortality Weekly Report* noted that ten people contracted amebic dysentery following colonic irrigation; seven eventually died.

According to the American Colon Therapy Association, today's conditions are sanitary and greatly improved. This should reduce the major health risks of infection and death that can occur under nonsterile treatment conditions. However, other problems may result from colonic irrigation, including enzyme imbalance, perforation of the colon, and general weakening of the body, a special concern for patients with cancer and other serious illnesses.

The ideology on which colonic irrigation is based—that dried food and toxins remain stuck inside the walls of the colon—is not physiologically accurate. According to scientists, toxic material does not remain and putrify in the colon, ready to cause bodily toxification. A 1987 report published by the American Medical Association's Council on Scientific Affairs summarized data that debunked the notion of autointoxication. Today's trained medical clinicians similarly do not believe in the idea of autointoxication.

What It Can Do for You

Proponents recommend colon therapy as a preventive measure for healthy people and to help cure disease. There are exceptions: advocates do not recommend colon therapy for individuals with ulcerative colitis, diverticulitis, Crohn's disease, hemorrhoids, or intestinal tumors.

Colonic irrigation is not used in mainstream medicine. However, enemas, which do not reach up into the colon, are used to relieve some cases of constipation and to enable some radiologic evaluations (the barium enema is an example).

Those who seek colon therapy should be alert to the cleanliness of the office and the equipment. If the equipment is not properly sterilized, or if disposable applicators are not used, the very real danger of infection exists. If you want to try colon therapy, discuss it first with your physician in case there are medical or other contraindications.

Colon therapy received widespread publicity when tabloids revealed that a British princess received it two or three times a week (much too frequently, says the American Colon Therapy Association, which recommends twice yearly as a maintenance regimen). However, it is not used in mainstream medicine.

Where to Get It

The American Colon Therapy Association is in San Antonio, Texas (210 366-2888). Many states have societies of colonic hygienists or colon therapists. For information about intestinal diseases and nutrition, contact:

✦ Gastro-Intestinal Research Foundation
70 East Lake Street, Suite 1015
Chicago, IL 60601
Telephone: (312) 332-1350

✦ Intestinal Disease Foundation, Inc.
1323 Forbes Avenue, Suite 200
Pittsburgh, PA 15219
Telephone: (412) 261-5888

✦ Centers for Nutrition Policy and Promotion
1120 20th Street NW, Suite 200
North Lobby
Washington, DC 20036
Telephone: (202) 418-2312

Enzymes are protein molecules that are essential to the numerous chemical reactions that continually occur in the body. Specialized enzymes play a major role in digestion by breaking food down into chemical components that can be absorbed and used by the body. Digestive enzymes are produced by the salivary glands in the mouth and by the stomach, pancreas, and small intestine.

Enzyme supplements are used in mainstream medicine to treat people with serious illnesses such as cystic fibrosis, Gaucher's disease, and celiac disease—rare illnesses with strong genetic components that typically arise early in life and interfere with the normal digestive process. Healthy individuals do not require additional enzymes for normal digestion. The body's digestive system, as well as enzyme-containing plants consumed in the diet, provide all the enzymes needed.

Proponents of enzyme therapy, however, believe that digestive enzyme supplements play a broader role than just digesting food, and that food digestion is part of treating illnesses, even those that are unrelated to the digestive process. Proponents claim that enzyme supplements can be used specifically to fight illness. By aiding digestion, supplements help the body restore health and well-being, they say.

Advocates claim that supplemental pancreatic enzymes help the immune system fight disease. This idea stems from the work of Dr. Edward Howell in the 1920s, who believed that consuming large amounts of enzyme-containing raw foods would allow the body to use up less and "store up" more of its own enzymes. This, in turn, would enable the body to digest more efficiently and to absorb more nutrients.

What It Is

Enzyme therapy involves the consumption of enzyme supplements, available in health-food stores. They consist of enzymes extracted from plants and from animal organs, including protease (which digests protein), amylase (which digests carbohydrates), lipase (for fats), and

The lack of consistency between enzyme therapy and scientific understanding of digestion and enzyme activity has not deterred the continuing promotion and use of enzyme therapy to maintain general well-being and to treat many types of illnesses.

Pancreatic enzymes were first applied as cancer treatment in 1902 by John Beard, an English embryologist. Later, German researchers used enzymes to treat patients with multiple sclerosis, cancer, and viral infections.

Beard and the German researchers claimed therapeutic successes, although neither they nor anyone else has conducted scientific studies or produced research data that support their claims.

cellulase (which digests fiber). Usually the supplements are sold as capsules.

Advocates recommend consumption of supplemental enzymes between meals, claiming that at this time the enzymes can be absorbed directly into the bloodstream to assist the immune system to clear viruses and other infections instead of remaining in the intestinal track to aid digestion.

What Practitioners Say It Does

Proponents claim that enzyme supplements, while aiding digestion and healing digestive ailments, also can cure sore throats, hay fever, ulcers, and viral illnesses. The use of pancreatic enzymes to treat cancer remains unproven and controversial.

Beliefs on Which It Is Based

Enzyme therapy is based on the belief that "more is better." The human body naturally produces enzymes that aid digestion and assist absorption of nutrients into the bloodstream. Proponents of enzyme therapy recommend increasing the amount of enzymes above the level produced by the body.

Research Evidence to Date

Aside from personal reports printed and promoted by manufacturers of enzyme supplements, there is no scientific evidence to substantiate proponent claims for enzyme therapy. Enzyme products have been reviewed by consumer groups and by the Food and Drug Administration (FDA).

In 1985, *Consumer Reports* published an article entitled "Foods, Drugs, or Frauds?" The article stated that numerous companies promoting enzyme therapy were violating federal laws with false advertising and distributing incorrect information. Later that same year, the FDA launched its own investigation. One company, Enzymatic Therapy, was ordered to stop producing its "Research Bulletins," because the publications contained false information. In 1991, after six years of inspection, the FDA began injunction proceedings because the company continued to make false claims about the nonexistent "healing power" of enzyme supplements. In late

1992, a court order banning promotional material with unproven claims was issued.

What It Can Do for You

Enzyme therapy consists of bogus products with nonexistent benefits. Enzyme supplements are broken down by the body just as other proteins are, and enzymes are changed into chemical substances that the body can absorb.

Where to Get It

Information about digestive disorders and treatment are available from:

◆ The American Dietetic Association, which maintains a toll-free nutrition information hot line: (800) 366-1655.
◆ Digestive Disease National Coalition
711 Second Street NE, Suite 200
Washington, D.C. 20002
Telephone: (202) 544-7497
◆ National Digestive Diseases Information Clearing-house
Two Information Way
Bethesda, MD 20892-3570
Fax: (301) 907-8906

28 ✑
Metabolic
Therapies

Metabolic therapy is based on the theory that disease is caused by accumulations of toxic substances in the body. Treatment, accordingly, aims to eliminate the toxins. It is believed that this will enhance immune function, which in turn will assist the body to restore itself to health. Metabolic therapies vary from practitioner to practitioner, but typically include the same basic components: a special diet; high-dose vitamins, minerals, and other dietary supplements; and detoxification with coffee enemas or irrigation of the colon (see Chapter 26).

The development of metabolic therapy is attributed to Max Gerson, a physician who emigrated from Germany to the United States in 1936. After successfully treating patients with lesser illnesses, he expanded metabolic regimens to patients with cancer. Today cancer is the most common illness treated with metabolic therapy.

The Gerson Clinic, along with many others specializing in metabolic therapies, is still active in Tijuana, Mexico. Tijuana is close enough to the United States to draw patients who can afford the fees, and outside U.S. borders to avoid potential problems such as the use of unproven products. At least seven metabolic clinics or hospitals dot the hills around Tijuana, which remains a hub of activity in metabolic therapy. Metabolic clinics run by physicians have opened recently in the United States.

Variations on Gerson's method have been developed by several followers, such as William Donald Kelley, an orthodontist by training; biologist Harold Manner, Ph.D.; Ernesto Contreras, M.D.; and others. All had clinics in Tijuana. Nicholas Gonzalez, M.D., practices his own version of metabolic therapy in New York City, where research to evaluate the potential benefits of his regimen is underway.

What It Is

Metabolic treatment typically is initiated in the clinic, where patients remain on an inpatient basis. A diagnosis is made using conventional blood tests as well as unscientific tests such as hair, urine, and blood crystal-lization analysis. Because all diseases are believed to result from the same underlying disorders, treatment is similar regardless of diagnosis.

As an example of a metabolic regimen, the Gerson diet is essentially vegetarian. Raw-liver juice, formerly part of the therapy, was abandoned by contemporary Gerson therapists in 1989 because of contaminants found in much commercially available liver. Each patient is given about twenty pounds of fruit and veg-etables a day, typically consumed in the form of pure carrot and apple juices.

Detoxification, another major component of metabol-ic therapy, consists of coffee enemas every four hours. The enemas are claimed to stimulate the excretion of bile from the liver and rid the body of toxins.

Meals with predominantly natural and organically grown foods, plus nutritional supplements, are eaten to strengthen the immune system. Meditation, prayer, and additional alternative therapies such as bioelectric stim-ulation may be used to aid the fight against cancer and other illnesses.

What Practitioners Say It Does

Proponents of metabolic therapy take the position that they address the underlying cause of disease, which they say is a buildup of (unspecified) toxins. They fault mainstream medicine for treating only "symptoms." Advocates believe that cancer and other illnesses stem from toxicity-induced disruption of the immune system, which creates an internal environment susceptible to the development of disease. The toxins are said to come from chemicals in food, water, and air pollutants. Eliminating the internal toxins is believed essential to rejuvenating the body's immune system, which in turn is thought to allow self-healing from cancer and other ill-nesses to occur.

Beliefs on Which It Is Based

Gerson's therapy was based on the view that malig-nant growths result from metabolic dysfunction within cells. This was to be countered by diet and detoxifica-tion. The use of coffee enemas was based on German medical tradition in the 1920s, when rectally induced caffeine was found to stimulate the production of liver bile in laboratory animals. Gerson believed also that an imbalance between sodium and potassium in each cell also contributed to the development of cancer. Therefore, his therapeutic diet excludes sodium and provides abundant potassium (see Chapter 8).

Research Evidence to Date

Contemporary research does not substantiate the beliefs and practices of metabolic therapy. The American Cancer Society strongly urges people diagnosed with cancer not to seek metabolic treatment unless and until data indicate that it is safe and effective. The National Cancer Institute awaits data from Gonzalez as he treats cancer patients with his own metabolic regimen.

What It Can Do for You

Electing metabolic therapy or any unproven treatment over mainstream medicine may cause patients to lose valuable time in receiving treatment with proven benefits. The discomforts and financial costs of receiving an unproven treatment far from home are substantial, especially when there is no evidence that the therapy may be beneficial.

Some components of metabolic therapy may pose serious health risks. Continued use of enemas, for example, will cause the colon's normal function to weaken, worsening problems with constipation. Coffee enemas remove potassium from the body and could cause potentially fatal electrolyte imbalances. Some metabolic clinic diets, used in combination with enemas, risk dehydration.

Where to Get It

For information regarding cancer and mainstream cancer treatment, contact:
+ American Cancer Society
  1599 Clifton Road NE
  Atlanta, GA 30329
  Telephone: (800) ACS-2345 [227-2345]

+ National Cancer Institute Hotline
  National Institutes of Health
  9000 Rockville Pike
  Bethesda, MD 20205
  Telephone: (800) 4-CANCER [422-6237]

Information about metabolic therapy is available through:

+ Gerson Clinic
  P.O. Box 430
  Bonita, CA 91908
  Telephone: (619) 267-1150
+ Gerson Research Organization
  7807 Artesian Road
  San Diego, CA 92127

29
Neural Therapy

When your dentist numbs an area of your mouth before drilling to fix a cavity, he or she uses an anesthetic injection such as novocaine. Anesthetic injections also are used to control severe localized pain. Neural therapists also inject anesthetics like novocaine or lidocaine in various parts of the body, but they do so for different reasons.

They believe that such numbing injections remove blockages that inhibit the body's electrical energy flow, and that the anesthetic travels throughout the body to heal illnesses. The initial conceptual basis for neural therapy was provided by the Russian physiologist Ivan Petrov. He theorized in 1883 that the nervous system influences all organic functions.

His beliefs seemed to explain a situation that occurred in 1940, when a physician named Ferdinand Huneke injected novocaine into the shoulder of a patient suffering from "frozen shoulder," a condition involving a stiff and painful shoulder unable to be moved normally. The patient's shoulder did not respond to the medication, but an old scar from a previous leg injury began to itch. On a hunch, the doctor injected the scar with novocaine. The patient's shoulder healed immediately. Although this reaction is not recorded in the annals of science, it is known in alternative medicine as the **Huneke phenomenon**, where it is assumed to indicate that the scar had become an "interference field," a blockage of energy flow that caused the frozen shoulder.

Combining inferred energy interference and local injections of anesthetics, Huneke and his associates established a new treatment process they called neural therapy.

What It Is

Neural therapy is the injection of anesthetics into various sites such as nerves, acupuncture points, glands, scars, and trigger points (points that produce a sharp pain when pressed). The injections are said to remove blockages, or interference fields, thus restoring electrical conductivity throughout the body and enabling healing to occur.

Medical Conditions Treated by Proponents of Neural Therapy

Allergies	Circulatory	Glaucoma	Inflammatory eye	Prostate diseases
Arteriosclerosis	disorders	Hay fever	disease	Sinusitis
Arthritis	Colitis	Headache	Kidney disease	Skin diseases
Asthma	Depression	Heart disease	Liver disease	Sports injuries
Back pain	Dizziness	Hemorrhoids	Migraine	Thyroid disease
Bladder	Ear problems	Hormonal	Muscle injuries	Ulcers
dysfunction	Emphysema	imbalance	Postoperative	Whiplash
Chronic pain	Gallbladder disease	Infertility	recovery	

Practitioners locate interference fields by charting the patient's health history. The history includes past illnesses, injuries, and treatments, as well as symptoms of current problems. Evaluation of this information enables development of a treatment plan, and the injections begin. Some patients may receive only one injection; others may require a series of several.

What Practitioners Say It Does

Although neural therapy is all but unknown in America, it is commonly used by physicians in German-speaking countries. Local injections of anesthetics are given for pain control or to stimulate adaptive physiological functions. Proponents make it clear that neural therapy can treat many medical conditions. It is applied most commonly, however, to treat chronic pain.

Beliefs on Which It Is Based

Proponents believe that most illnesses are caused by interruptions in the body's electrical system. Somewhere a breakdown of communications between cells occurs. When communication is impeded, what is known as an interference field develops. Any previous illness or injury may create an interference field, causing disturbances in the electrical (communication) system at the trauma site and anywhere else in the body.

It is believed that anesthetic injections allow the body's electrical system to regain its normal energy flow, thus restoring health. Proponents admit they do not fully understand how this occurs or how neural therapy works. Various theories have been proposed. One suggests that injecting the anesthetic into the interference site allows "blocked" cells to regain lost energy and resume communications. In turn, this alleviates the medical problem currently experienced by the patient.

Research Evidence to Date

Other than proponent literature, there is no scientific evidence to support neural therapy and its concepts. Researchers in Germany indicate that anesthetic injections do effectively reduce pain, but the mechanisms behind the remaining claims for neural therapy await investigation.

What It Can Do for You

Proponents of neural therapy do not recommend it for genetic diseases, nutritional deficiencies, mental conditions (other than depression), or end-stage chronic diseases. Clearly, neural therapy should be avoided by anyone allergic to anesthetics. Because there is no relevant scientific research, neural therapy cannot be recommended for any medical condition.

Patients receiving injections of anesthetics for conventional pain control should receive this treatment under the care of a licensed neurologist who specializes in pain management.

Where to Get It

For more information regarding the treatment of chronic pain, contact:

✦ National Chronic Pain Outreach Association, Inc.
7979 Old Georgetown Road, Suite 100
Bethesda, MD 20814
Telephone: (301) 652-4948

✦ American Chronic Pain Association, Inc.
P.O. Box 850
Rocklin, CA 95677
Telephone: (916) 632-0922

Oxygen—without it we cannot live for more than a few minutes. We breathe it in from the air, and our red blood cells carry it through the bloodstream to nourish organs and tissues. Can oxygen, as produced by ozone and hydrogen peroxide—two oxygen-rich chemicals—cure serious diseases such as cancer and AIDS? Advocates of a group of therapies known variously as hyperoxygenation, bio-oxidative therapy, oxidative therapy, oxymedicine, and ozone therapy, claim that it can.

What It Is

By whatever name, oxygen therapies involve administering ozone or hydrogen peroxide into the body for the purpose of treating disease. Most oxygen molecules in the atmosphere are composed of two atoms. When this oxygen, known as O_2, collides with single atoms of oxygen under the right conditions, a three-atom molecule of oxygen, known as **ozone,** or O_3, is created.

We are familiar with the term *ozone* from media reports about the ozone layer. The ozone layer is in the upper atmosphere, approximately thirty miles above the earth's surface. Because of its chemical structure, ozone is capable of absorbing certain forms of radiation from the sun. If this radiation were not absorbed but instead passed through to the earth's surface, plant and animal life as we know it could not exist on earth.

In the lower atmosphere, however, *ozone* can be a health hazard. Here it is a product of chemical reactions between sunlight and nitric oxide from car and factory emissions. If the ozone concentration in the air gets too high, it can irritate eyes and lungs and aggravate the problems of asthmatics and others who suffer breathing difficulties.

Ozone is not an accepted or proven medical therapy. However, advocates promote it for use in several ways. It is administered intravenously, through injection into muscle or skin, or by infusion into the rectum or vagina. Some practitioners draw small amounts of blood from the body, place the blood in a machine that infuses ozone into it, and then pump the ozone-rich blood back into the patient.

Hydrogen peroxide (H_2O_2) is composed of two atoms of oxygen and two atoms of hydrogen. It is formed when water reacts with a single atom of oxygen. Hydrogen peroxide, used in mainstream medicine for wound cleansing and disinfection, is applied to the skin only. In contrast, advocates of oxygen therapy promote regimens involving internal delivery of hydrogen peroxide. Most ozone or hydrogen peroxide treatments involve injection of diluted solutions of ozone and hydrogen peroxide in doses given over a period of one to several weeks.

What Practitioners Say It Does

Advocates of oxygen therapies claim that it treats and can cure many diseases. One contemporary advocate lists over thirty illnesses that hydrogen peroxide and ozone therapy are said to treat effectively. This list includes such serious conditions as asthma, emphysema, AIDS, chronic fatigue syndrome, Alzheimer's, and certain cancers.

Ozone and hydrogen peroxide produce oxygen atoms with facility. Ozone is unstable and splits easily into two atoms: one stable oxygen molecule and one atom of oxygen. Hydrogen peroxide also will split into a molecule of water (which consists of two hydrogen atoms plus an oxygen atom) and one atom of oxygen. These single oxygen atoms, according to oxygen therapy advocates, provide oxygen that the body uses both to prevent diseases from starting and to fight diseases already present in the body.

Beliefs on Which It Is Based

Advocates of oxygen therapy believe that disease is caused by microorganisms that thrive in low-oxygen environments. The microorganisms are said to thrive because they are less complex in terms of evolutionary development than normal body cells are, and therefore they require less oxygen. Lacking adequate oxygen, microorganisms in body tissues are thought to be able to spread and cause disease.

These microorganisms are implicated in heart disease, cancer, and arthritis, among other illnesses. According to oxymedicine advocates, our bodies can become depleted of oxygen by pollutants, poor diet, stress, and other causes. When ozone therapy is administered, oxygen levels are raised. Elevated oxygen levels are believed to destroy the disease-causing toxins and microorganisms.

A major theoretical foundation for oxygen therapy is the work of Otto Warburg, M.D., winner of the Nobel Prize for medicine in 1931 (for elucidating the chemistry of cell respiration). Warburg observed that cancer cells have lower respiration rates than normal cells. He postulated that cancer cells therefore grow better in a low-oxygen environment, and that introducing higher oxygen levels could retard their growth or kill them.

However, researchers now understand that cancer cells' lower-than-normal respiration is due to the fact that tissue surrounding cancer cells receives less oxygen because it has fewer blood vessels feeding it. Ozone and other oxygen therapies have not been found useful against cancer and are not used as mainstream cancer treatments.

Research Evidence to Date

A study of ozone therapy for use against HIV and hepatitis is now underway at several major medical centers in Italy. Conducted under the supervision of a research hematologist based in New York, the trial applies a new technology for delivering ozone. This involves generating ozone as a thin film, which is assumed to keep the concentration low enough to protect healthy cells, but high enough to destroy HIV or hepatitis viruses. This is believed feasible because the membranes of viruses are simpler than those of normal cells and therefore easier for ozone to attack. The results of this multisite study will not be available for several years. Although its theoretical basis appears sound to scientists, there is no way to know until the research concludes whether this treatment will be effective in human beings.

What It Can Do for You

Potential medical uses of both ozone and hydrogen peroxide have been explored for over a century. In the 1920s, hydrogen peroxide was used to treat the flu. In the 1940s it was studied in animal tests for possible use against carbon monoxide poisoning. For these uses, hydrogen peroxide was shown to be ineffective or much less effective than other available therapies. Hydrogen peroxide currently is applied in medicine only to cleanse and disinfect wounds and in dentistry as an irrigating agent in treating root canal problems and gum disease.

Similarly, ozone has been studied for its potential medical benefits since the nineteenth century. In recent times it has been investigated for possible use against AIDS. Ozone showed an ability to inactivate the HIV virus in blood and serum in laboratory experiments. However, follow-up studies in people with AIDS have been disappointing, failing to show that ozone had an effect against the disease. Treatments that appear promising in the laboratory are not always effective in humans.

As of this writing, hydrogen peroxide and ozone are not accepted as useful therapies for serious disease. Hydrogen peroxide can be harmful, causing toxic reactions if taken internally in excessive amounts or as an undiluted preparation.

Where to Get It

Patients with AIDS or cancer should not consider oxygen therapies as either alternative (first-line) or adjunct (complementary) therapies. Because ongoing research continually brings new treatment information about cancer and AIDS, people seeking the latest information should contact the National Cancer Institute or the National Institute of Infectious Diseases and Allergy at the National Institutes of Health (NIH):

+ National Cancer Institute Hotline
  Telephone: (800) 4-CANCER [422-6237]
+ National Institute of Allergy and Infectious Diseases
  Telephone: (301) 496-5717
+ Public Health Service Hotline
  Telephone: (800) 342-2437

In the early part of this century, as sanitation improved and medicine and microbiology advanced, infectious diseases, which had been a major cause of early and pervasive death, dwindled as threats to public health. More people lived to old age. This meant that more people were in a position to develop chronic illnesses such as heart disease and cancer. Indeed, the incidence of such illnesses increased as large segments reached ages at which chronic conditions become prevalent.

Attention focused on chronic illnesses such as heart disease, diabetes, and cancer. In 1974, a "war on cancer" was declared in the United States. A commitment was made to finding improved methods of detecting, treating, and ultimately curing and preventing cancer. Billions of dollars and decades of effort on the part of government, academia, and industry poured into this effort over the years. Despite impressive gains in the treatment and understanding of cancer and its genetic underpinnings, cancer remains a major killer.

The absence of a cure for cancer enabled those outside of mainstream medicine to develop alternate explanations of cancer's cause along with treatments based on those explanations. Such treatments are unproven and alternative. Shark and bovine (cow) cartilage therapies are current popular examples. They are promoted not only as cancer therapies, but also to treat disorders such as osteoporosis and other bone and joint problems. They remain unproven but under investigation as potentially promising agents against cancer.

What It Is

Cartilage is the part of the skeletal system composed of elastic, translucent tissue, most of which converts to bone as animals grow to adulthood. However, some cartilage remains in areas such as the ears, nose, and knees. Because sharks have no bones, cartilage is the primary component of their skeletal system. Cows, of course, do have bones, but their skeletal system also contains cartilage.

Patients using bovine cartilage as a cancer treatment typically take a 3-gram dose by mouth three times a day.

Shark cartilage requires much higher dosages, typically 60 to 90 grams each day either orally or by enema. Patients often take shark cartilage by enema because of the high doses required and because shark cartilage tastes very bad, often inducing nausea in the amounts recommended. A typical regimen of bovine cartilage treatment costs $160 per month, versus $700 per month for shark cartilage. Because shark and bovine cartilage treatments are unproven treatments for any illness, they are available only in health-food stores and through the mail as food supplements. As such, they are not reviewed or regulated by the Food and Drug Administration (FDA) for safety or effectiveness.

What Practitioners Say It Does

Advocates claim that shark and bovine cartilage can reduce tumor size, slow or stop the growth of cancer, and help reverse bone diseases such as osteoporosis.

The popularity of shark cartilage can be traced back to a 1992 book entitled *Sharks Don't Get Cancer*, by I. William Lane, Ph.D. (Sharks do, by the way, get cancer, including cartilage cancer, but the incidence of cancer in sharks is low.) In his book, Lane claims that sharks avoid cancer because of substances in their cartilage. In 1993 a popular television program featured a small study conducted in Cuba suggesting that shark cartilage shows promise as a cancer treatment. The promotion of shark cartilage for bone diseases began shortly after new government regulations allowed food supplements to be promoted without FDA review and without proof of efficacy.

Beliefs on Which It Is Based

The idea that bovine or shark cartilage may have an effect in cancer treatment actually is based on one of the most promising areas of contemporary cancer research: angiogenesis. **Angiogenesis** refers to a process necessary to the growth of tumors. In order to remain alive, tumors, like all cells and body parts, require fresh supplies of blood and oxygen. If a tumor has no blood vessels to "feed it," it will not continue to grow but will die. Scientists are now working to discover effective ways of halting the blood supply to tumor cells.

There is a protein in cartilage that can inhibit angiogenesis in test-tube laboratory research. However, this does not mean that cartilage can fight tumors in the human body. In addition to the difficulties involved in translating lab results into research on live patients, cartilage has other potential problems. The most serious problem is that the active ingredient in shark cartilage is too large to be absorbed into the blood stream from the digestive tract, and therefore is excreted from the body before it can actually perform any function. This is what happens to the shark cartilage promoted for human use.

Bovine cartilage molecules are small enough to be absorbed into the body. Advocates believe that bovine cartilage may work by inhibiting the growth of tumors or by boosting the immune system. The leading advocate and researcher of bovine cartilage believes that substances in bovine cartilage, known as polysaccharides, work to stimulate the immune system. He bases that belief on the fact that other kinds of polysaccharide compounds have both immune-stimulating and anti-cancer activity in humans. If researchers prove this to be true, it might also explain the mechanism by which shark cartilage might work if its molecules were small enough to be absorbed into the bloodstream.

Research Evidence to Date

Several studies have examined the effectiveness of shark and bovine cartilage against cancer. However, none adhere to scientifically accepted principles of research design, so their results are not meaningful. The results have not even been published.

The United States National Cancer Institute initiated a study of shark cartilage in 1994. It was halted because each batch of cartilage sent by advocates to be used in the experiment was contaminated. Very few studies have been published on the effects of bovine cartilage against cancer. One was reported in 1985 by John Prudden, M.D., the leading researcher of bovine cartilage. It involved thirty-one patients, of whom 61 percent had complete tumor remission and 90 percent had some response to a bovine cartilage preparation. Patients with many types of cancer were included in the study, weakening its results. Prudden, while continuing to study and administer bovine cartilage treatment, has not published further work on its effectiveness.

What It Can Do for You

There is no firm evidence that cartilage treatment is effective against cancer, and there is no evidence whatsoever about cartilage as a treatment for osteoporosis or any bone disease. Given the available evidence or lack of evidence, it is difficult to recommend shark or bovine cartilage even as adjuncts to conventional cancer treatments. Certainly they are not recommended as first or main cancer therapies.

In fact, the sponsor of an Internet cancer information service who himself used bovine cartilage as a cancer patient strongly cautions against taking bovine cartilage instead of conventional cancer treatment. However, bovine cartilage is not terribly expensive, and it does not appear to interfere with other medications.

Where to Get It

Both bovine and shark cartilage, available through mail-order catalogs and health-food stores, are sold in capsule or powder form under a variety of brand names. Keep in mind that neither product is regulated by the FDA and has not been approved or inspected for effectiveness or safety.

REDUCING PAIN AND STRESS THROUGH BODYWORK

The therapies in this section may be perceived as body-mind, as opposed to mind-body, medicine. From Part III we saw that mind-body therapies such as hypnosis, biofeedback, and meditation claim to improve physiological and psychological well-being through manipulating or training the mind. In contrast, the therapies described in this part share the belief that health problems can be alleviated or prevented, and well-being improved, by manipulating all or parts of the body. This is accomplished through specific exercises or manual manipulation by others.

The therapies in this part are distinguished by the fact that they are not invasive. Some, however, such as chiropractic, attempt to alter the position of bones or muscles through manipulation. Other approaches focus on the body surface with the somewhat different goal of simply relieving tense muscles rather than bringing about permanent realignment. Yet other approaches, such as yoga, represent systems of movement, practiced and perfected through diligent effort, that aim to realign the body or promote relaxation.

Most therapies in this section, although not all, can be practiced on your own, following instruction from a teacher. Thus most are inexpensive, and some are free after an initial training period. Many are safe and gentle, with few side effects. All, however, must be evaluated individually, because the potential for harm or injury from a practice performed incorrectly does exist. Also, people with potentially precluding circumstances should check with their physicians before starting bodywork: these include people with certain physical conditions such as fragile bones;

The Versatility of Bodywork

Bodywork techniques seem to help people regardless of whether they are healthy or ill.

Bodywork can reduce problems such as stress or depression among those coping with serious illness.

Used to enhance well-being in those who are ill, the same techniques can be part of a wellness-oriented lifestyle for those who are disease-free.

infants with still pliant bones; and those with certain illnesses or open wounds.

In general, proponents of the therapies in this part do not claim to cure disease. Compared to other groups of alternative therapies, the claims made for most bodywork regimens are less sweeping and more focused on enhancing well-being than on healing illness. Indeed, most bodywork techniques are presented, even by their advocates, as complementary therapies designed to augment conventional curative techniques for those with illness, and to increase relaxation, help reduce stress, and otherwise enhance quality of life in those who are healthy.

Massage therapy and the Alexander technique, for example, promise to increase well-being by relieving muscle tension and altering poor habits of posture and movement, respectively. Others promise to speed relief from self-limiting conditions such as headaches.

Where do these therapies come from? Almost all epochs and cultures have produced bodywork methods. The origins of some techniques, such as yoga and tai chi, are so distant in time as to be not clearly understood. The typically ancient beginnings of these therapies, not surprisingly, are usually associated with primitive, simplistic theories to explain their effectiveness. These theories are rarely supported by mainstream science, and sometimes the two sets of theories conflict with each other.

It is possible, however, for a therapy to be effective even if ideas about how it works are incorrect. For example, tai chi may induce relaxation by means similar to those of traditional exercise rather than through the claimed improvement in circulation of the life force *qi* (or *chi*, pronounced "chee"), but that does not lessen its ability to promote relaxation.

Over time, practitioners from some bodywork systems split into various camps, so that variations in emphasis often exist within the same therapy. Some chiropractors, for example, restrict their practices to spinal manipulation, which is associated with chiropractic's earliest ideas, while others incorporate additional therapies and approaches into their work. Similarly, several advanced students of Rolfing split off over the years, modifying, extending, and discarding aspects of the original approach, and adding their own insights, to develop new methods of bodywork. There are also different schools of tai chi and yoga, each practicing a variation on the main theme.

Some bodywork methods stem from or are closely related to other systems of alternative medicine. Indeed, some may be perceived as the physical expressions of those alternatives. For example, tai chi is based on principles similar to those behind traditional Chinese medicine, and practitioners of traditional Chinese medicine often practice tai chi themselves and prescribe it for others. Acupressure recognizes acupuncture's system of pressure points, but uses manual pressure instead of needles to achieve its effects. Yoga and other physical methods are part of a broad philosophical and healing worldview, of which bodywork is just one part.

The mechanisms of action known or hypothesized for these therapies may be placed into one of three categories: The most common explanation is that they increase or unblock "energy flow" throughout the body; less often they are said to correct misalignment in the whole body or in a part; and very rarely they are said to be consistent with principles of physics or chemistry.

Therapies such as acupressure, tai chi, and reflexology are based on the assumption that the body contains energy that flows through it. These therapies claim to strengthen and balance this energy flow, although they differ in their explanations of the source and path of this flow. For example, acupressure and tai chi rely on the ancient concept of *qi*, a hypothesized energy force that travels through the body along paths known as meridians. Reflexology, by contrast, does not have a name for its energy force. The flow to various organs is believed to be stimulat-

Complementary, Not Alternative

Claims made for bodywork techniques usually are appropriate.

There are exceptions, however. Some practitioners promote complementary therapies, such as no-touch healing or craniosacral therapy as cures for cancer and other major illnesses.

Buyer beware!

ed by pressing parts of the foot that are said to be linked to these organs.

Some therapies begin with the hypothesis that the body has an ideal alignment, that misalignment causes discomfort or problems, and that therapy can restore ideal alignment. For example, the Alexander technique claims that the body's ideal posture involves the head, neck, and spine aligned in a specific way. Although related therapies share the principle that the body's misalignment causes problems, they differ on the issues of how and where the body becomes misaligned, and what should be manipulated to correct the problem. Chiropractic relies on manipulation of the spine, while Rolfing attempts to realign the **fascia**, the tissues that cover the muscles and connect them to the skeleton.

In contrast, hydrotherapy uses established effects of heat and cold on the circulatory system to explain its benefits. It becomes alternative (rather than complementary) only when practitioners make claims that cannot be proved or explained by these mechanisms, or when it is applied in dangerous ways, such as to treat kidney and liver problems.

There are many other systems of bodywork in addition to those discussed in this section. Most use some combination of hands-on work and movement exercises and share the same beliefs that lie behind most bodywork regimens: that emotional trauma can cause long-term physical tension; that bad habits of movement can be replaced with good to reduce muscular tension; and that an energy force exists that can be strengthened and balanced through bodywork. Some additional approaches are summarized below. Most were developed in the past fifty years.

Aston Patterning A student of Ida Rolf (see Chapter 39), Judith Aston added movement exercises and rearranging clients' environments to Rolfing's deep-tissue manipulation. Like Rolfing, Aston patterning seeks to change habits of movement and reduce muscular and skeletal pain and tension.

Bioenergetics Developed by Alexander Lowen, M.D., bioenergetics is based on the belief that repressed emotions cause muscular tension, and that a combination of bodywork and psychotherapy can relieve both muscular tension and repressed emotions.

Feldenkrais Method This system, known as "Awareness through Movement," is designed to make patients' patterns of movements easier and more efficient.

Hellerwork Developed by Joseph Heller, a former president of the Rolf Institute, Hellerwork adds movement exercises and counseling to Rolfing's manual methods. Hellerwork involves eleven 90-minute sessions during which patients are taught to move more efficiently in ways that are natural to their body type.

Myotherapy Manual pressure is applied to "trigger points," which are said to be unique in each patient's body. Trigger points, caused by trauma, are claimed to cause muscular tension and discomfort, problems said to be eliminated by several sessions of myotherapy.

Polarity Therapy Based on principles of traditional Chinese and Ayurvedic medicine, polarity therapy was developed by Randolph Stone, a chiropractor, osteopath, and naturopath. While the client lies on a massage table, the practitioner gently places both hands on the client. Their energy is said to comingle and the client's energy blockages to be relieved.

Rosen Method Developed by Marion Rosen, a physical therapist, this approach is based on the concept that repressed emotions cause muscular tension. Practitioners gently massage the patient's body, attempting to reduce muscular tension as patients' emotions are discussed.

Rubenfeld Synergy Ilana Rubenfeld, a former music conductor and student of the Alexander technique and the Feldenkrais method, also developed a combination of talk therapy and hands-on work. Practitioners locate and touch spots of tension on patients' bodies while patients describe their emotional problems.

Shiatsu An ancient Japanese system of massage, shiatsu involves gentle pressure to the meridians postulated by traditional Chinese medicine to unblock and balance *qi,* the body's hypothesized flow of energy.

Trager Psychophysical Integration (Tragerwork) Developed by Milton Trager, M.D., the goal of Tragerwork is to change habits that limit movement ability and cause muscular pain or tension. Using a system called "Mentastics," it aims to make movement more pleasurable and effective.

Acupressure

Acupressure is the pressing of specific acupuncture points in order to relieve pain and stress in a particular area or part of the body. Pressure can be applied by one's own or another's fingers, or, in response to particular problems, by a button on a wristband. Acupressure probably was a formalized outgrowth of the natural human tendency to stroke, massage, or press the body until pain is relieved.

One can imagine the process becoming increasingly sophisticated over the centuries, as pressing specific points on the body was found, perhaps by group consensus, to relieve distress in particular areas. In turn, acupressure seems to have given rise to a more technological (albeit still ancient) variation—acupuncture.

Although **shiatsu** often is assumed to be the same as acupressure, it is not. They are similar in that they both involve applying pressure to acupoints. However, shiatsu is new and focuses on prevention rather than healing. It is a modern outgrowth of ancient acupressure.

What It Is

Acupressure is acupuncture without the needles. A type of massage, it involves placing very firm finger pressure for a few minutes on an **acupoint**, which is a specific place on the skin. More than 100 acupoints dot the lengths of hypothesized meridians (channels) that run vertically from head to toe throughout the body. The acupoint to be pressed is determined according to which energy channel is blocked and therefore causing the problem.

There are fourteen meridians, twelve of which are bilateral—that is, the same points exist on both sides of the body. The two remaining meridians, which are unilateral, run along the midline of the body. Meridians are the invisible interior channels through which qi (life force or vital energy) is believed to travel throughout the body (Figure 17). (These pathways are not consistent with any biological systems known to Western science, such as specific nerves or blood vessels.) Each acupoint is believed to control particular body organs or functions.

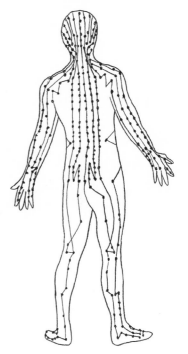

Figure 17 Hundreds of acupuncture points line the body's hypothesized twelve head-to-toe meridians. Pressure on a point relieves pain and stress in often distant associated areas of the body.

What Practitioners Say It Does

According to Chinese lore developed thousands of years ago, acupressure is said to remove trapped energy, assist the free flow of the life force, and dissipate problems in areas of the body associated with a particular meridian.

Claims made for acupressure vary by practitioner. Some claim that the technique successfully treats obesity, arthritis, and pain and improves blood circulation. Others believe that acupressure can function as an effective preventive measure, maintaining health through the promotion of balance in body organs and systems. The claims of others, especially those in mainstream medicine, are more modest, tending to stress acupressure's ability to relieve pain in many people.

Beliefs on Which It Is Based

Acupressure stems from the ideas on which traditional Chinese medicine (see Chapter 3) rests, and is rooted in the beliefs and assumptions of that ancient healing system, including the flow of *qi* throughout the body. When *qi* meets no blockages and can move smoothly, balance and harmony are said to exist in the body, a state equivalent to health. Conversely, when the flow of *qi* is blocked, internal imbalance results, a condition that is tantamount to illness.

The fundamental belief behind acupressure, then, is that pressing certain points on the body, called acupoints, can remove energy blocks along relevant meridians, returning balance to the body and enabling healing to occur.

Research Evidence to Date

Studies have assessed acupressure's effectiveness with several problems, including morning sickness in pregnant woman, postsurgical nausea and vomiting, headaches, motion sickness, and backache. Research results are mixed.

In the acupressure/acupuncture system, nausea is believed to be controlled by a small area on the inside of the wrist called the P6 acupressure point. Pressing that point is believed to assist vital energy flow along the meridian that leads to and controls the nausea center, and thus relieve the symptoms.

Headache?

Some people obtain relief by pressing the soft area between thumb and forefinger, using the thumb and forefinger of your other hand.

Press hard for a few minutes. It may work, and it won't do any harm.

One study of pregnant women found no relief of nausea. Another scientific investigation, however, found that P6 acupressure reduced nausea for some women but did not lessen vomiting. In a study of visually induced motion sickness, sixty-four subjects were randomly placed in four groups. Those who received P6 acupressure reported feeling less nauseated than the others, and their motion sickness symptoms decreased. A study of women after gynecologic surgery found that those who received P6 acupressure made fewer requests for antivomiting medication. Also, a separate investigation involving a similar group of patients who were in surgery for six to eight hours found that P6 acupressure effectively prevented nausea and vomiting.

The ability of acupressure to reduce headaches was shown in a study reported twenty years ago. This research project followed 500 patients for two years, and found that acupressure techniques were reasonably effective in relieving headache pain. The acupoints used in efforts to eliminate headache are located on the hands and feet as well as the head and neck. The particular point or points pressed depend on the type and location of the headache. Research suggests that applying pressure to specific acupoints also can reduce chronic backache.

What It Can Do for You

Some people benefit from acupressure, although research is very limited and fails to explain the mechanisms by which acupressure works. The rationale for its occasional effectiveness may be the relaxation and comfort that results from hands-on massage, the pressure that results in the release of endorphins (which are the body's natural painkillers), or some other cause. Although very hard or deep pressure may be somewhat painful, acupressure is not invasive and may be worth a try.

Some obvious precautions are in order. Acupressure should not be used as the only treatment for a chronic problem or for serious injury or illness. In these cases, a licensed physician should be consulted. Acupressure should be avoided near the abdominal area in pregnant women and near varicose veins, wounds, sores, or bones that may be broken.

Acupressure Versus Other Kinds of Bodywork

Most bodywork involves manipulating muscle groups or the entire body.

Acupressure involves pressing on a single point, often distant from the pain, believed related to the aching area on the basis of ancient Chinese concepts of energy flow and blockage.

Where to Get It

Typically, information about acupressure and its practitioners can be found in the Yellow Pages of the telephone book or in resource directories under "bodywork," "acupuncture," or "massage."

The Acupressure Institute in Berkeley, California (510 845-1059), and the American Oriental Bodywork Association in Syosset, New York (516 364-5533) can also provide you with information.

⁀33
Alexander Technique

Frederick M. Alexander, pioneer of the Alexander technique, depended on one of the oldest human tools, simple self-observation, to develop his bodywork system. The Alexander technique is the legacy of one man's effort to heal himself.

Alexander was an Australian actor, born in 1869. While performing on stage one night, he lost his voice. He periodically suffered additional episodes of voice loss on stage, and the problem threatened to end his acting career. Visits to physicians resulted in prescriptions for rest and medications, but these did not solve the problem.

Alexander began to observe himself in a mirror. He noticed that when he practiced his roles he lowered his head and tensed the muscles in his neck, which he concluded led to strained vocal cords. Over several years of observation and effort, he corrected these postural habits, and his problem cleared up. He began to help others with posture or movement problems, eventually moving to London and starting a program to teach his methods. He ran that program until his death in 1955.

Alexander developed methods to change the way his body moved when engaged in everyday activities such as standing, sitting, walking, and speaking. His technique promises those who study it increased relaxation, a greater sense of well-being, and better overall body function.

What It Is

The goal of the Alexander technique is to correct bad habits of posture and movement that, over time, can lead to poor posture, excessive muscle and body strain and tension, and inefficient ways of moving.

The method usually is taught one-on-one, but group classes may be held as well. During class, which typically lasts thirty to forty-five minutes, students go through several different types of exercises. The teacher may have the student go through everyday activities such as walking or sitting. As the student sits, for example, the teacher gently uses his or her hands to move parts of the body that are strained or tense in order to begin teaching the student how to sit in the proper way.

At the same time, the teacher gives verbal directions about how to relax and properly align parts of the body. Students may spend part or all of a class lying down, as the teacher continues the process of giving directions and redirecting muscles with his or her hands. Students are asked to keep the exercises in mind outside of class.

There are no set number of lessons required to complete Alexander technique training. Rather, students study until they feel that they have learned what they need to know.

Perhaps due to the origin of the method, the Alexander technique is particularly popular with actors, dancers, and musicians, and classes in it are often taught at performing arts schools. Certified teachers complete a 1,600-hour training program over a three-year period. In the United States there are seventeen independently run teacher-training programs approved by the North American Society of Teachers of the Alexander Technique (NASTAT), and about 600 certified teachers.

What Practitioners Say It Does

According to advocates, the Alexander technique can correct habits of poor posture and movement that can lead to muscle strain, pain, and imbalance in the body. The Alexander technique is used by healthy people as well as by those suffering from muscular and skeletal strain, tension, or chronic pain induced by problems with posture or movement.

For those in pain, the technique can help alleviate muscular strain and tension that cause or exacerbate this pain. For the healthy, it can improve awareness of the body and enhance efficiency of movement and posture. Also, it is said to improve physical coordination, increase well-being, and promote relaxation. The goal is to teach the correct way to move the whole body, not to work with one area or part of the body. In the process of learning how to move correctly, pain alleviation is possible.

According to Alexander advocates, the technique is distinguished from other systems of bodywork and from medical therapies by Alexander's theory of proper body alignment and by the particular methods he developed.

Beliefs on Which It Is Based

Alexander believed that optimal alignment of the head, neck, torso and spine exists when posture and movement are correct. In this alignment, the head rests comfortably at the top of the spine, and the spine is neither compressed nor incorrectly curved. When the body is perfectly aligned, its muscles are relaxed and ready for movement.

Alexander and his current followers believe that his exercises, properly practiced, enable students to unlearn those habits of movement and posture that cause difficulty, and to learn proper posture and movement that put the body back into alignment. Alexander believed that bad habits develop very slowly, starting in childhood, so they often go unnoticed until later in life.

Research Evidence to Date

Alexander teachers have written a great deal about the technique. There are even several journals devoted to the Alexander method. Articles discuss the use of the Alexander technique in clinical settings with pregnant women, and for those suffering from voice loss or lower back pain. These publications, however, as is true for many alternative regimens, are descriptive rather than investigative. They do not contain research data that evaluate the approach, and therefore they have not been published in the mainstream medical literature.

An exception is a 1992 study. It found that people who received twenty weekly training sessions in the Alexander technique increased their respiratory function, whereas respiratory function did not improve in a group of control subjects.

What It Can Do for You

The Alexander technique has prospered in terms of its spread and the number of teachers and students it attracts. However, despite many anecdotal testaments to its efficacy, its claims have not been validated through research. Those who are curious about it or want to see whether it will relieve muscular pain or tension may want to try it. The technique is gentle and not likely to cause harm. And it may indeed work for you, bringing pain relief, relaxation, and the more efficient body function it claims to bestow.

People with chronic muscular pain or joint difficulties should consult with their primary caregiver to make certain that it will not interfere with any treatment or exacerbate a condition.

Where to Get It

There are several organizations of Alexander teachers in the United States. The largest is:

✦ NASTAT
3010 Hennepin Avenue South
Minneapolis, MN 55408
Telephone: (800) 473-0620
Internet: http://www.life.uiuc.edu/jeff/nastat.html

This organization can provide names of certified Alexander teachers in your area. There are many books about the technique, including four written by Alexander himself.

Chiropractic may be the most commonly used alternative therapy in the United States today. There are an estimated 50,000 chiropractors, the third-largest group of health practitioners in the country. Some chiropractors are called "mixers" because they combine chiropractic with exercise. Those who depend on chiropractic alone are identified as "straight" practitioners.

Founded in the 1890s by a grocer and mystic healer in Davenport, Iowa, the movement got its start when D. D. Palmer believed he had restored a patient's hearing by thrusting his hand on the patient's thoracic vertebra where he believed the cause of the deafness was located. Palmer subsequently opened the first school for chiropractic training, which he based on the idea that the spine plays a major role in health and disease.

Although originally developed to treat a rather narrow spectrum of problems, primarily low back pain, some practitioners today believe that chiropractic can cure cancer and other major as well as lesser diseases. Although modern colleges of chiropractic have broadened their training to include clinical sciences, laboratory experience, and clinical practice, there is potential danger in chiropractors accepting patients with serious conditions that they have not been trained to understand and treating them with manipulation.

Chiropractors are licensed in all fifty states, and their services are covered by Medicare and many health insurers.

What It Is

Chiropractic (from the Greek meaning "done by hand") is a belief system that depends primarily on manipulation of the spine to correct medical problems. The chiropractor analyzes the condition of the spine through X rays and palpation, looks for irregularities or misaligned vertebrae that may interfere with the function of the bundle of nerves inside the vertebrae, and attempts to manually readjust vertebrae that cause nerve interference and pain. The specific medical diagnosis usually is not important to chiropractors, who focus instead on correcting the cause of the imperfect function and rely on the body's greater intelligence to repair the disease.

Typically, practitioners take a medical history and perform a physical examination. They focus on muscle strengths and weaknesses, range of spinal motion, structural abnormalities, and variations in posture. Some practitioners also may examine electrical activity of the nerves and muscles. Frequently (too often, according to some physicians), X rays of the spine are taken to look for irregularities. Chiropractors also seek to identify the seat of illness through manual procedures.

Chiropractors treat by manipulating the spine by hand, using high-velocity, low-force recoiling thrusts, or perhaps rotational thrusts with hands or elbows, and apply appropriate pressure to the spinal area identified as the source of pain or disease.

Spinal manipulation is not a new idea in medicine. It was practiced by priest-healers of ancient Egypt, and for centuries in one form or another by Asian healers. Throughout the Middle Ages in Europe, it was used along with herbal medicines to treat patients. In more modern times, osteopathic medicine began to grow in popularity at about the same time Palmer was developing his concepts of chiropractic. **Osteopathy** initially relied on spinal manipulation in a manner similar to chiropractic.

What Practitioners Say It Does

Back pain is one of the most frequently reported health problems. It is said that, sooner or later, back pain will affect three out of four Americans. It ranks second only to the common cold as a reason for doctor's office visits. Low back pain is the most common problem brought to chiropractors, although headache, shoulder pain, neck pain, sports and workplace injuries, tension, and carpal tunnel syndrome (pain, weakness, numbness, or tingling in the arm or hand) also are frequently treated by chiropractors.

Today, chiropractors do not necessarily limit their work to musculoskeletal problems. Most believe they are able to successfully treat ailments no matter where they occur in the body or what their cause. Thus, many chiropractors treat heart disease, prostate and impoten-cy problems, allergies, and epilepsy. Some seek to estab-lish primary-care practices in family medicine or pedi-atrics. They believe that these efforts are appropriate because the chiropractic belief system credits the spine with a major role in virtually all problems of health and disease.

It should be noted that, although chiropractors focus their therapies on the spine, not all critical nerve sys-tems are accessible for manipulation along the spine. Cranial nerves, which affect the face, including the eyes, ears, tongue, and throat, bypass the spine because they are contained within the cranium and are not accessible to manual manipulation.

Beliefs on Which It Is Based

Chiropractors are taught that the human body has an innate ability to heal itself, and that it seeks to maintain a state of homeostasis, or balance, among all its body systems and organs. The nervous system influences all other systems in the body; therefore, it is viewed as the focal point in treating health problems. Because the brain sends energy to all parts of the body through nerves contained in the spinal cord, it is reasoned that displaced or dislocated vertebrae could interrupt energy flow along the nervous system, causing a physical blockage of neural transmissions, a condition Palmer labeled **subluxation**.

Proper therapy for correcting subluxations is thought to involve quick thrusts or "adjustments" to the spine, plus various types of manual manipulations to correct the aberrant relationship between bone and nerve. Uncorrected, subluxations are thought to allow disease and bodily malfunctions to occur.

Today, some chiropractors define subluxation more broadly, calling it a complex involvement of nerves, muscles, and spinal movements. Some believe the word appropriately refers to joint dysfunction. Despite dis-agreement among chiropractors over the role and defin-ition of subluxation, the belief that disorders of the spinal structure underlie disease remains intact. Chiropractors also believe that health problems can be identified and treated through manual manipulation.

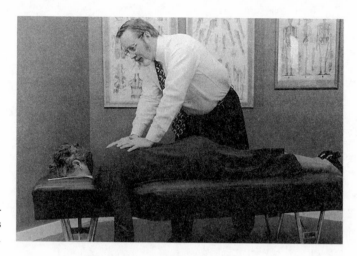

Figure 18 It is important to understand the appropriate applications of chiropractic therapy.

Research Evidence to Date

Although the chiropractic profession has conducted rigorous research for many years, little of it has been published in responsible medical journals. A 1992 Rand Corporation study examined reports of twenty-two clinical trials involving chiropractors and other types of practitioners using spinal manipulation. The report concludes that manipulation is effective in varying degrees for treatment of patients with some types of low back pain.

A study called the *Magna Report,* published in Canada in 1993, states that chiropractic manipulation is better on three counts than traditional medical care for low back pain: it is more effective, safer, and less expensive. The *Magna Report,* however, has been criticized, with dissenters claiming that its conclusions exceeded information on which they were based.

What It Can Do for You

Manipulation of the spine by a chiropractor usually makes people feel better. Manipulation may correct a dislocation and solve the problem of chronic lower back pain. Chiropractic therapy may improve posture, relieve headaches and tension, and successfully address other discomforts generally eased by manipulation or massage (Figure 18). Similar benefits may be obtained by treatments given by physical therapists.

Because their training is often at odds with modern

medical understanding, particularly in anatomy and physiology, you may not want to consider using a chiropractor as a family physician or to treat illness or disease. Research evidence does not support chiropractic claims that cancer or other diseases can be cured with spinal manipulation.

Where to Get It

There are approximately 50,000 chiropractors currently practicing in the United States. All fifty states and the District of Columbia license chiropractors, and practice typically is regulated by chiropractic boards.

Chiropractors are listed in the Yellow Pages of most telephone directories. Although the American Chiropractic Association lists some 15,000 members, the most convenient local resource is your telephone book. Chiropractors usually are not bashful about advertising. Some even offer special deals for initial visits.

There are at least eight national and international chiropractic associations. A major source of information and printed material is the American Chiropractic Association in Arlington, Virginia (703 276-8800).

35 ⋞⋟

Craniosacral Therapy

Many if not most alternative therapies have come from ancient cultures in distant parts of the world. Craniosacral therapy is different because it is relatively new and it developed in the United States. This therapy relies on some basic ideas that are not proven by conventional science. Moreover, pediatricians writing in medical journals have expressed concern about the harmful effects of craniosacral therapy on children and infants.

Craniosacral therapy was created in the early 1900s by Dr. William G. Sutherland, who trained in Kirksville, Missouri, at the first school of osteopathy. An expanded version of craniosacral therapy was developed in the 1970s by the osteopathic physician John Upledger at the Upledger Institute in Florida. He and the thousands of health-care professionals who attend his training programs annually focus on releasing stresses in the skull and the membranes surrounding the brain.

What It Is

Craniosacral therapy is a spin-off of chiropractic and osteopathic medicine. Unlike those broader fields, however, it applies a lighter touch with its hands-on therapy and focuses only on the craniosacral system—the bones of the head, spine, and pelvis (Figure 19). This approach differs from chiropractic also because its goal is not to adjust the relationship between the musculoskeletal and nervous systems, but rather to increase the flow of cerebrospinal fluid. Gentle massage is applied to eliminate obstacles to the free flow of cerebrospinal fluid. The practitioner may also emit no-touch healing energy to the client. Each craniosacral massage session can last from thirty minutes to an hour or more.

What Practitioners Say It Does

Craniosacral therapists believe that their treatment normalizes, balances, and eliminates obstructions in the central nervous system, the immune system, and other systems throughout the body. Relieving obstructions to the normal rhythm of cerebrospinal fluid flow is said to allow the central nervous system and the entire body to function properly and healthfully.

Therapy is recommended for infants and children as well as adults. Craniosacral therapists believe that the difficulties and stresses of the birth process can distort growing cranial tissues, so they attempt to align the cartilage and membranes of the skull. They claim success for a broad variety of childhood problems, including hyperactivity, cerebral palsy, and earache. (Please see the "Word of Warning" box on page 224). In the adult, craniosacral therapy is said to cure brain and spinal injury, seizures, menstrual dysfunction, chronic pain, autism, and many other ailments. Recently, a leading craniosacral therapist reported curing a woman of breast cancer.

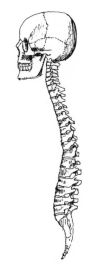

Figure 19 The craniosacral system includes the skull bones, the spine into the pelvis, and the surrounding cerebrospinal fluid.

Beliefs on Which It Is Based

The fundamental premise of craniosacral therapy is that manipulation of the head can correct abnormalities in cerebral membranes, which in turn can influence the pressure of cerebrospinal fluid. Craniosacral practitioners believe that they can restore a patient to health by manipulating his or her craniosacral system. The craniosacral system includes the skull (cranium), the spine down to its tail end (the sacral area), and the pelvic bones. It also includes the membranes that surround these bones and the cerebrospinal fluid that bathes the brain and spinal cord.

Like many alternative therapies, craniosacral therapy is built on the view that illness is caused by blocked channels of energy or bodily fluids. Treatment, therefore, aims to release blockages and restore free flow. Proponents believe that the bones of the skull move in rhythmic patterns. However, the idea that the bones of the adult skull move at all, let alone in patterns, is not consistent with any scientific understanding of human anatomy.

Research Evidence to Date

Research on craniosacral therapy has produced mixed results. No definitive evidence is available to document its effectiveness or even to support the basic premises on which the therapeutic approach is based. Those who practice this type of therapy claim many successes. But according to Upledger and colleagues in a report to the NIH Office of Alternative Medicine, successes have not been documented in formal studies. Anecdotal reports and personal histories are offered instead.

Important questions about how and whether craniosacral therapy works remain to be answered. Proponents say it is possible to measure craniosacral rhythms and changes in these rhythms. They also claim that craniosacral abnormalities are closely related to disease. However, medical researchers find that craniosacral rhythms are difficult to measure reliably, calling into question the notion that rhythms actually exist.

The basic concepts behind craniosacral therapy—that moving the bone plates of the skull will result in better health and elimination of some disorders—is not consistent with what is taught in medical schools around the world. According to scientific understanding of skeletal anatomy, the bones of the skull fuse together firmly by the time a child reaches age two, and cannot be moved by hands pressing the head.

Therefore, if anatomical science is correct, it is impossible to influence underlying membranes or cerebrospinal fluid pressure by moving bones of the skull, because these bones do not move (although craniosacral proponents believe they do). Furthermore, mainstream specialists explain that merely lying down on your back produces more change in the pressure of cerebrospinal fluid than does the manipulation of craniosacral bones.

What It Can Do for You

Even if craniosacral therapy does none of the things it claims to do, it still can be helpful. It can decrease stress, release muscle tension, and enhance well-being. Prolonged hands-on attention, the opportunity to rest comfortably in a relaxed position while someone ministers to your body, the benefits of human touch for up to an hour or more—these and other aspects of the therapy are heart-warming, muscle-relaxing, and beneficial, even if there is no evidence that the procedure cures illness. However, serious problems may result from using this procedure with children whose skull bones are not yet fused.

Where to Get It

Most practitioners of craniosacral therapy are osteopathic or chiropractic doctors with additional training in the craniosacral method. These doctors as well as their professional associations can provide referrals.

The following specialty groups provide information and referrals as well as craniosacral manipulations:

+ Cranial Academy, Indianapolis, Indiana (317 879-0713).
+ Upledger Institute, Palm Beach Gardens, Florida (407 622-4706).

36 ⤳
Hydrotherapy

Our planet and our bodies are mostly water. We cannot live for more than a few days without it. Water has been a part of medical practice from the beginning of civilization to the present day, and great healing powers have been ascribed to it, as illustrated by clichés such as the "fountain of youth" and "healing waters."

The Romans built bathhouses across the extent of their empire. Scandinavian countries are famous for their saunas. Following the practice throughout Europe, resorts in the United States were developed around the mineral waters of Hot Springs (Arkansas), Warm Springs (Georgia)—where Franklin Roosevelt often went to seek relief from his polio-caused physical disabilities—as well as many other sites. Today, water-based therapies are used throughout conventional, complementary, and alternative medicine to treat wounds, injuries and burns, to facilitate physical rehabilitation, and to promote relaxation (Figure 20).

What It Is

The use of water as a medical treatment is known as hydrotherapy. Because hydrotherapy encompasses so many different approaches, any particular form should be evaluated along several dimensions. First, is it part of conventional or unconventional medicine? One of the largest and most widespread complementary uses of hydrotherapy comes in the form of spas and bathhouses. In many countries, resorts have developed around natural springs. These resorts typically were created in the belief that minerals in the spring water could aid the healing of disease. Spas sometimes offer other forms of hydrotherapy, such as mud or seaweed baths.

Second, is it applied externally or internally? Examples of external hydrotherapies include ice packs to reduce the swelling of sprained ankles, warm water to irrigate and cleanse wounds, and whirlpool baths for physical rehabilitation. Internal hydrotherapies include administering fluids to dehydrated patients. An example of an unproven and possibly dangerous hydrotherapy is **colonic irrigation** (see Chapter 26).

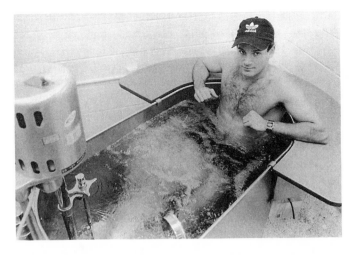

Figure 20 Hydrotherapy in the form of a hot shower or whirlpool bath (shown here) relaxes muscles and reduces stress. It is also recommended for sports injuries.

Third, what is the state or temperature of the water? It could be solid (ice), cold or hot liquid (water), or gas (steam). In Japan, Scandinavia, Turkey, and other countries, public bathhouses have been an integral part of community life for centuries. At the end of the workday, people gather and either soak in heated water (**steam bath**) or sit in a steam-filled room (**sauna**) for twenty minutes or so. Sometimes, periods of time in a sauna are alternated with periods of time out in the cold air or even quick dips in icy water or snow.

Fourth, what is the duration or pressure of the water used in the treatment?

Fifth, what is the stated and desired purpose of the treatment?

Finally, is the hydrotherapy self-administered or administered by a practitioner?

Home-based hydrotherapy systems, such as **hot tub**s, Jacuzzis (**whirlpool baths**), and home saunas, offer the relaxation benefits of public baths. They often include showerhead or handheld devices that provide water massage.

Another form of hydrotherapy is the **sitz bath**, where the pelvis is immersed in a tub of warm water. The sitz bath is said to offer relief from pelvic-area soreness and abdominal and other ailments.

What Practitioners Say It Does

Hydrotherapy has several major functions in conventional medicine. The first is hygienic, involving the cleaning and irrigation of wounds or burns to enable additional treatment or prevent infection. Pain relief is another important role, as in the case of cold compresses for headaches or hot water packs for muscle pain. Hydrotherapy, including the use of ice packs, is applied to ease the effects of minor injuries, such as ankle sprains. Internal body temperature can be regulated with water, both to reduce fevered body temperature or raise abnormally low temperatures caused by excessive exposure to cold.

Hydrotherapy is used also for physical rehabilitation and exercise. Conducting therapy or exercising in water can be more effective and cause less strain and trauma to the skeleton and joints than is true for land-based therapies.

In complementary medicine, hydrotherapy provides relaxation and symptom relief from many ailments, as listed later in this chapter. In alternative medicine (therapies promoted for use instead of mainstream conventional care), hydrotherapy is cited as a potentially curative therapy. Colonic irrigation is an example. Such unproven methods may involve exposing the body to extremes of temperature through water or through cleaning it internally with water—procedures claimed to increase health by detoxifying the body and restoring it to health.

Beliefs on Which It Is Based

Many hydrotherapies are based on well-known, documented physiological effects either of water itself or of heat or cold delivered through water. **Heat-based hydrotherapies** rest on the fact that heat dilates (expands) blood vessels, which increases circulation in the area being heated. Increasing the blood supply to muscles with the application of heat, for example, can relieve pain.

Cold-based hydrotherapies work according to an opposite mechanism. Cold constricts blood vessels, reducing circulation to that area of the body. Application of ice or cold packs is useful to reduce swelling. Physical rehabilitation activities in swimming pools are based on the fact that water is more protective of the skeletal system and offers more resistance than air, which enables muscles to work harder while protecting bones and joints.

Research Evidence to Date

Ice packs, hot compresses, and sinking into a warm tub are good examples of tried-and-true, self-help, water-based techniques that work on a host of common problems. Some are described in the following section. Water immersion removes weight from joints and facilitates motion and exercise. In addition, hydrotherapy is a major component of therapy for hospitalized patients with severe burn injuries, and heat therapy is a proven method for skin diseases.

Conversely, a review of the medical literature indicates that hydrotherapy for more serious and prolonged conditions than those listed below is not effective. For example, hydrotherapy did not reduce pain, swelling, immobility, or other problems in careful studies of patients with osteoarthritis of the hip or rheumatoid arthritis, patients after knee- or hip-joint surgery, or following ligament, cesarean, and other gynecologic surgical procedures.

What It Can Do for You

The following self-help remedies have been found safe and useful:

- **Abdominal cramps, irritable bowel syndrome** A heating pad or hot-water bottle applied to the abdomen usually helps.
- **Arthritis and bursitis** Use gel or ice packs for pain resulting from overactivity; apply heat for swollen, tender, hot joints; and take a hot shower or bath to relieve stiffness and pain. Alternating ice and heat, ten minutes for each application, helps bursitis.
- **Breast soreness from pregnancy**, **menstruation, benign discomfort** Heating pads work for some women, cool-water compresses for others, and some achieve comfort by alternating hot and cold applications. (See your physician for any new lump.)
- **Carpal tunnel syndrome** For this condition, caused by long-term, repetitive motions of hands and wrists, use ice packs.

Reducing Pain and Stress through Bodywork

- **Colds, laryngitis, sore throat** Humidity helps these and related ailments. Stand in a hot shower, use a humidifier, try a steam bath, or place your face over a bowl of steaming water with a towel draped over your head, forming a mini–steam bath.
- **Headaches** Hot compresses or heating pads are the usual treatment, but some people get more relief from cold compresses applied to forehead and neck.
- **Hemorrhoids** A sitz bath—sitting in warm water with knees raised—reduces pain and shrinks swollen veins.
- **Hives** Cool baths, cold compresses, or an ice cube rubbed on the hives can all be helpful.
- **Insomnia** A warm bath a few hours before bed can induce drowsiness.
- **Insect stings** Ice cubes or an ice pack are helpful, but some people feel better with applied heat.
- **Menstrual cramps and endometriosis** If a heating pad does not help, some women find relief with cold packs.
- **Muscle aches and pains and swelling** Use ice packs twenty minutes on, twenty minutes off for several hours or a day.
- **Stress** Soaking in a hot tub restores proper circulation, relaxes the body, and reduces stress.
- **Sunburn and other minor burns, bumps, bruises, sprains** Apply ice water or ice compresses, or apply a cloth dipped in cool water.

Although hydrotherapy has many benefits and applications, some caveats are in order concerning various forms of its use:
- Cases of bacterial diseases infecting users of improperly cleaned public and private whirlpools and hot tubs have been reported in the medical literature.
- Excessively hot water can cause burns and other problems; ice applied directly to skin for more than a short time can damage tissues.
- Excessively cold water can harm people with circulatory disorders.
- Be wary of outlandish claims made for the curative value of any hydrotherapy.
- Particularly regarding internal hydrotherapies, be aware of possible side effects or harm from excessive water

temperature, pressure, or amount of liquid infused.

- Colonic irrigation can cause perforation of the colon. Furthermore, serious and even fatal internal infections have been caused by this procedure in practices that fail to sterilize equipment.

Where to Get It

- ✦ Conventional practitioners often prescribe hydrotherapy as part of physical therapy and other treatment regimens.
- ✦ For self-administered hydrotherapies, check your phone book for local spas, health clubs, and YMCAs that have whirlpool or sauna facilities.
- ✦ Hydrotherapy equipment can be purchased for use in the home.
- ✦ Those interested in alternative forms of hydrotherapy may want to consult a naturopathic doctor, as forms of hydrotherapy often are included in naturopathic approaches to healing (see Chapter 6).

37 ⬎

Massage

Massage today is considered a respectable and viable complementary technique. Modern massage is used not only as a form of stress reduction and muscle relaxation, but also as an adjunctive treatment for patients in hospitals and retirement centers.

The history of massage is four to five thousand years old. The renowned 2700 B.C. Chinese text, *The Yellow Emperor's Classic of Internal Medicine*, recommends that "breathing exercises, massage of the skin and flesh, and exercises of the hand and feet" be used to treat paralysis, chills, and fever. Early Egyptian tomb paintings display therapeutic massage, clearly indicating its application in that part of the ancient world as well.

As massage evolved, Per Henrik Ling, a nineteenth-century physician in Sweden, developed **Swedish massage**, considered to be the most commonly practiced massage technique today in the United States. His method was based on gymnastics, physiology, and techniques borrowed from China, Egypt, Greece, and Rome.

What It Is

Massage is the use of various manipulative techniques to move the muscles and soft tissues of the body. Swedish massage consists of five specific types of strokes:

1. **Effleurage** is a long gliding stroke done with the whole hand or thumb.
2. **Petrissage** involves kneading and compression motions.
3. **Friction**, the most penetrating of the movements, consists of deep circular movements made with the therapist's thumb pads or fingertips.
4. **Vibration** involves applying a very fine, rapid shaking movement.
5. **Tapotement** consists of a series of quickly allied movements using the hands alternately to strike or tap the muscles.

Therapists may use some or all of these techniques during a massage session depending on the area being worked, the training level of the therapist, and the pref-

Eastern versus Western Massage

The philosophies of Eastern and Western massage, both of which are popular, differ importantly. Eastern thought stresses restoration of the body's energy, while Western belief focuses on the importance of relaxing muscles and tissues.

Both techniques, however, share the goal of assisting the body's natural healing ability. Massage helps individuals reduce stress as well as recover from physical problems.

The Alternative Medicine Handbook

erence of the client. A massage session may last from thirty to sixty minutes. Cost generally ranges from $30 to $75.

The room in which massages are given contains a sheet-covered massage table, which is similar to an exam table in a doctor's office. Typically the room is softly lit and bathed in low, soothing music. The client is partially or totally undressed and covered with a sheet or towel. The cover is moved and then replaced from each part of the body as it is massaged (Figure 21). It is important that clients tell their therapists what they expect and what they are comfortable with. Explaining any physical ailments also is necessary.

In some cities, minimassage is available to workers during their lunch breaks, providing quick relief of stress in a brief period of time.

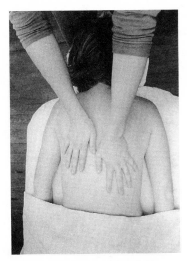

Figure 21 Massage is one of the most universally beneficial of complementary therapies.

What Practitioners Say It Does

Massage has important emotional and psychological benefits. It relaxes muscles, which in turn reduces stress. Massage is helpful not only in reducing the feeling of being stressed, but also in treating problems exacerbated by muscle tension, such as insomnia, headaches, and backache. Massage can also help in the treatment of high blood pressure, arthritic and rheumatic pain, asthma, colds, constipation, depression, and even diabetes.

Beliefs on Which It Is Based

In an ancient Greek text, Hippocrates described massage as an effective therapy, especially for sports and war injuries. Although historically, as with Hippocrates, massage was used as a medical treatment, it has been proven over time to be effective therapy for the mind as well as the body. Many advocates of massage refer to the relevance of "healing touch." This contact between the massage therapist and client is said to sooth the soul and the mind.

Massage therapy is based on an understanding of its physiological effects. When muscles are overworked, waste products such as lactic acid can accumulate in the muscle, causing soreness, stiffness, and even muscle spasm. Massage improves circulation, which increases

Derivation

The word *massage* comes from *massa*, an Arabic word meaning "to stroke."

blood flow, bringing fresh oxygen to body tissues. This can assist the elimination of waste products, speed healing after injury, and enhance recovery from disease.

Research Evidence to Date

Massage is beginning to receive the research attention it deserves, and the medical community increasingly uses massage therapy as a complementary treatment for various illnesses and with different subject groups. A 1995 medical journal reported that infants and children with various medical conditions who received massage therapy had lower anxiety levels and got well sooner. Infants with HIV (human immunodeficiency virus, which causes AIDS) who received massage did much better than those who did not receive it. Massage also was found to reduce anxiety in children and adolescents under psychiatric care.

Another study documented a reduction of blood pressure among elderly nursing home patients who were given back massage. Several articles in medical journals describe the relaxing benefits of massage therapy as a complementary treatment for patients with major illnesses such as cancer and heart disease. Research indicates also that massage therapy enhances quality of life.

What It Can Do for You

There is little question that people benefit both physically and mentally from massage therapy, and that massage promotes relaxation, releases muscle tension, and reduces stress. Massage therapy is all but universally helpful. However, it should be avoided if you have fever, acute inflammation, infection, phlebitis, thrombosis, or jaundice. You should not be massaged at the site of a recent injury. Individuals with chronic conditions such as arthritis, cancer, or heart disease should consult a physician before seeking massage therapy. Those who are healthy and wish to relax, reduce stress, and enhance their well-being should benefit from massage.

Where to Get It

The Yellow Pages of your local telephone book are a good source of information about local professional massage therapists. Books on massage include:

Giving a Massage at Home

1. Keep the lights low and the room warm.
2. Cover your partner with a sheet to avoid chilling.
3. A pillow under the knees or head may enhance comfort.
4. Use a pleasant, warmed oil on your hands to reduce friction.

+ *The Theory and Practice of Therapeutic Massage*, by Mark Beck (Milady, Albany, N.Y. 1994).
+ *Massage for Common Ailments*, by Sara Thomas (Fireside Books, New York, 1989).
+ *The Book of Massage*, by Lucinda Lidell (Fireside Books, New York, 1984).
+ *The Massage Book*, by George Downing (Random House, New York, 1972).

Although not all states regulate massage practices or license massage therapists, trained and duly qualified practitioners are widely available. The following organizations provide information about massage as well as referrals to qualified therapists:

+ American Massage Therapy Association
  820 Davis Street, Suite 100
  Evanston, IL 60201
  Telephone: (312) 761-2682
+ National Certification Board for Therapeutic Massage and Bodywork
  8201 Greensboro Drive, Suite 30
  McLean, VA 22102
  Telephone: (800) 296-0664 or (703) 610-9015
  Fax: (703) 610-9005

38 ⌒
Reflexology

Reflexology uses the foot as a map of the entire body. Pressing specific parts of the foot is believed to help heal problems in a related, albeit distant area.

Reflexology is not unique in adopting the idea that the sections of a single body part reflect each area of the entire body. Throughout the history of medicine, various attempts were made to use single body parts as diagnostic or treatment surrogates for the body as a whole. For example, whereas reflexology involves the feet, others use the iris of the eye. Their system of **iridology** claims to diagnose disease by relating each pie-shaped segment of the colored iris of the eye to a specific organ or part of the body. Although this technique remains somewhat popular today, iridology has been studied scientifically and proven useless. A nineteenth-century fad called **phrenology** attempted to map people's personalities according to the contours of their heads, linking bumps or prominent points on the skull to various character traits. Both Chinese and Ayurvedic Indian medicine use the tongue as a guide to diagnosing all manner of ailments in other body parts.

The ear is used as a surrogate for the entire body in aural acupuncture. In more modern times, the colon has been used as a map for other body areas, with each major illness said to reflect a disordered, perhaps too deeply creased, specific area of the colon.

Foot reflexology in the United States began with the work of William Fitzgerald, M.D., who practiced in Connecticut during the early years of the twentieth century. His technique was based on ancient practices that applied pressure to hands, ears, or feet to revive energy flow and bring about homeostasis (balance). Despite his area of expertise—he was an otolaryngologist, or eye, ear, nose, and throat specialist—his system uses none of these body parts, but rather the foot. The foot became a map of the whole body, each part relating to a specific body area.

Reflexology differs importantly from earlier attempts to use body parts as maps for the whole because it involves treatment as well as diagnosis. Fitzgerald theorized that the body is divided into ten equal zones that run from head to toe. With his system, which was initially called zone therapy, gentle pressure to certain points on the feet seemed to relieve pain in a particular area of the body.

In the 1930s, American nurse and physiotherapist Eunice Ingham developed detailed maps of the feet that included what she termed **reflex points** which link spots on each foot to specific body parts. Trial and error seemed to show that pressing the arch of the foot, for example, affected the inner organs. She also changed the name of the practice from zone therapy to reflexology.

Reflexology spread quickly throughout the United States and Europe. Most reflexologists working in the United States today have been trained in Ingham's method or that of another prominent reflexologist, Laura Norman. Ingham's nephew, Dwight Byers, currently president of the Florida-based International Institute of Reflexology, is considered the world's leading authority on the subject.

What It Is

Reflexology is a system of applying pressure to the foot. It is not massage. Instead, the practitioner's thumb, fingers, and palms apply pressure to specific reflex points on the foot. Reflexologists believe that each part of the foot relates to its own part of the body (Figure 22). By applying pressure to a reflex point, the corresponding body organ or area is affected.

Reflex points are on the soles, tops, and sides of the feet. The points on the right foot correspond to the right half of the body, and those on left foot correspond to the left half of the body.

Although people can perform reflexology on themselves after learning about the reflex points and pressure techniques, it usually is performed by a trained reflexologist. In a typical session, the patient lies on a massage table while the reflexologist gently massages each foot, and then begins treatment by systematically applying pressure to its reflex points.

Treatments last from thirty minutes to an hour. According to practitioners, patients may experience tingling sensations in areas of the body that correspond to reflex points as those points on the foot are pressed.

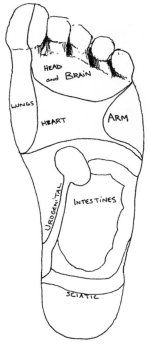

Figure 22 Reflexology uses the foot as a map of the body.

Reducing Pain and Stress through Bodywork

(The common basis of acupuncture and acupressure is clear here.) Reflexology is not painful.

What Practitioners Say It Does

Reflexology advocates believe that this approach can increase energy flow to the organs that correspond to the reflex points, and increase the vitality of those organs. By increasing the vitality of the internal organs, practitioners believe they can improve patients' health. They claim that reflexology can reduce stress and tension, improve circulation, eliminate toxins, and bring the body into a state of balance conducive to good health. These beliefs echo the vital-force concept that dominated the earliest ideas about health, illness, and physiological function.

Reflexology is recommended by proponents as a means of alleviating the symptoms of some chronic ailments, such as headaches, asthma, and bowel problems. It does not claim to cure illnesses.

Beliefs on Which It Is Based

There are two linked beliefs on which reflexology is based. One is that reflex points exist on the foot, and that these reflex points can influence health in distant organ systems and parts of the body to which they are linked. The second is that the body contains an invisible life force, or subtle energy, similar to the concept of *qi* (*chi*) in Chinese medicine and acupuncture (see Chapters 3 and 1, respectively), or *prana* in Ayurvedic or Indian medicine (see Chapter 2). Reflexologists believe that, by stimulating reflex points on the foot, they can unblock and increase the flow of this energy throughout the body.

Some reflexology advocates have offered hypotheses to explain the action of this subtle energy, or to interpret reflexology in physiological terms. They believe that energy travels from the nerve endings in the foot to the spinal cord, where it is disbursed to all parts of the body. Some advocates claim that reflexology releases endorphins, which are natural pain-blocking chemicals released by the brain. Others claim that reflexology detoxifies the body by dissolving crystals of uric acid that settle in the feet.

Research Evidence to Date

Research on reflexology in the medical literature is scant. A recent literature search found only two small pilot studies that have evaluated reflexology. These studies cannot be considered definitive. One shows that reflexology could contribute to headache relief, while the other reports that patients who received reflexology following gynecologic surgery needed less medication to maintain bladder function.

None of the beliefs and concepts on which reflexology is based, such as the idea of subtle energy, has been proven. The major underlying hypothesis—that pressure applied to the foot improves health—is also not documented.

What It Can Do for You

At this point, reflexology's claims to restore vitality and improve health, or to alleviate or control disease, must be considered unproven. As is true of various forms of bodywork, reflexology can promote relaxation and feelings of well-being. Although reflexology is not a proven method of treating disease, its potential relaxation benefits are obtained inexpensively and easily, especially because the technique can be self-administered. Also of great importance, reflexology is a gentle, noninvasive technique, free of side effects.

Where to Get It

There are many books about reflexology, and they are usually available in libraries and bookstores. Most contain reflex-point diagrams of the foot and explain how to apply reflexology's pressure techniques. Popular books include:

+ *Better Health with Foot Reflexology,* by Dwight Byers, (Ingham Publishing, St. Petersburg, Fl. 1987)
+ *Reflexology for Good Health: Mirror for the Body*, by Anna Kaye and Don Matchan (Wilshire Book Company, Hollywood, Calif. 1980)

The International Institute of Reflexology in St. Petersburg, Florida (813 343-4811), maintains and sells resources devoted to the technique, trains teachers, and keeps lists of reflexologists by geographic area.

39 ⬟

Rolfing

Structural Integration, or Rolfing, is a trademarked system of bodywork invented by Ida Rolf, Ph.D. (1896–1979). Rolf held a doctorate in biochemistry and physiology. In the late 1920s, the piano teacher of one of Rolf's children sustained a hand injury, which Rolf attempted to alleviate by giving the woman yoga exercises. This led to an interest in the relationship between body structure and function. After years of investigating body-oriented techniques such as yoga (Chapter 41), the Alexander technique (Chapter 33), and osteopathy, Ida Rolf developed Structural Integration. By the 1950s she was teaching the method. In 1970 the Rolf Institute was founded, and soon thereafter Rolf published books on the subject.

What It Is

Rolfing is an effort to align the body properly so that all segments—head, torso, legs, and so on—are correctly related to one another and aligned with gravity. This is accomplished by applying deep pressure to the **fascia**—the tissues that cover muscle fibers and internal organs, and help connect muscle to bone. Fascia play a key role in posture and overall support of the bones and skeleton (Figure 23). **Rolfers**, as they are called, believe that fascia become too solid and rigidly adhered, reducing the body's ability to execute smooth and full motion. Rolf believed that your emotional status reflects your structural imbalances.

Certified Rolfers use their fingers, thumbs, knuckles, and sometimes elbows and knees to press and thus manipulate fascia in all areas of the body. Rolfers aim to loosen the fascia so that its hold on muscle and bone will be released. Clients also execute a series of exercises geared to move their bodies more efficiently. People typically attend Rolfing sessions once a week for ten or more weeks. Each session lasts sixty to ninety minutes. Manipulation of the fascia is deepened at each successive session. Rolfing can be painful.

What Practitioners Say It Does

According to advocates, Rolfing can bring the body into

Rolfing Variations

Several of Rolf's students developed their own versions of bodywork based on Rolfing principles:

- Judith Aston created **Aston patterning**, a system of massage, movement education, and assessment of the client's living and working environment.
- Joseph Heller (not the novelist but the Rolf Institute's first director) developed **Hellerwork**. He believed that additional exercises were required to maintain changes initiated by manipulation of the fascia.

---

balance and alignment, working with rather than against gravity. As motion becomes easier, improved posture should result along with increased mobility, easier breathing, less stress, and more energy. Rolfing is said also to help reduce chronic pain, particularly resulting from problems such as lower back injury. Rolfing is not advocated as a curative treatment for disease. It is, however, felt to enhance one's general sense of well-being.

Beliefs on Which It Is Based

Structural Integration is based on two key premises. One is that the fascia can harden and thicken over time, throwing the body out of alignment with gravity. The other is the belief that a body out of alignment with gravity requires more effort and energy to move.

According to Rolf, the body ideally should be organized so that the centers of gravity of the head, shoulders, torso, and legs form a straight vertical line. When the fascia are relaxed and able to move, she believed, they can support this kind of structure.

Over time, however, poor posture, physical trauma, stress, emotional trauma, and disease can lead to the hardening and thickening of the fascia, causing the body to fall out of alignment. This is manifest in the drooping of head and shoulders, excess spinal curvature, and other postural defects. Structural Integration is said to manipulate the fascia so that they loosen and relax, restoring the body to its proper alignment.

Research Evidence to Date

A 1979 study found decreased levels of self-reported anxiety in patients who received Rolfing compared with patients who did not, and two small 1988 studies suggested that Rolfing could improve the angle of tilt in the pelvis. Controlled studies of Rolfing compared with other therapies or with no treatment are limited, and the claims made by Rolfing advocates are neither proven nor systematically examined.

What It Can Do for You

Whether Rolfing changes the body's alignment and whether realignment improves the efficiency of movement have not been formally studied, nor has the claim

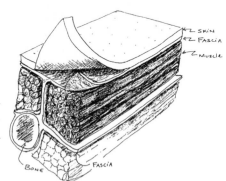

Figure 23 Rolfing massage manipulates the fascia, the connective tissues surrounding muscles and other body structures.

that Rolfing can improve well-being and quality of life.

On the other hand, Rolfing advocates do not claim to cure disease, and people have reported anecdotally that Rolfing improved their lives. It is possible that the Rolfing massage by itself, despite any associated discomfort or pain, may release tension, convey a sense of well-being, and/or bring other physical and emotional benefits associated with massage therapy in general (see Chapter 37).

Where to Get It

The Rolf Institute in Boulder, Colorado, teaches and certifies Rolfing instructors, and maintains records of where certified instructors are located. The institute will provide a list of certified Rolfers in your area:

+ Rolf Institute for Structural Integration
  205 Canyon Boulevard
  Boulder, CO 80302
  Telephone: (303) 499-5903
  Internet: http://www.rolf.org

Sources of information about related programs include:

+ Aston Training Center
  Box 3568
  Incline Village, NV 89450
  Telephone: (702) 831-8228
+ Hellerwork International
  406 Berry Street
  Mount Shasta, CA 96067
  Telephone: (916) 926-2500

Books about Rolfing and related practices include *Rolfing: The Integration of Human Structures*, by Ida P. Rolf (Harper & Row, New York, 1977).

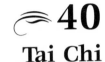

40
Tai Chi

Are you looking for a gentle exercise program that soothes your mind as it improves your body and works even if you are ill or elderly? Follow the daily example of millions of Chinese. Tai chi is an exercise regimen that uses movement, meditation, and breathing to improve health and well-being. Tai chi (pronounced "tie chee," as in *cheese*) probably originated as an exercise, like shadow boxing, to maintain agility among feudal warriors. It has become a daily exercise regimen for people old and young, sick and well, throughout China.

Although practiced in China for many centuries, tai chi has only recently gained popularity in the United States and other Western countries as an excellent general exercise technique. Tai chi is a more physically active form of *qigong* (see Chapter 20).

What It Is

Tai chi differs from the more intense and violent martial arts often depicted in films because its movements are gentle and deliberate. It relies more on technique than on physical prowess. Tai chi can be practiced by individuals of almost any age, size, or athletic ability, as proficiency does not require great strength or flexibility.

While practicing, students are reminded to pay close attention to their breathing. In tai chi, breathing is centered in the diaphragm rather than in the chest. Proper tai chi breathing is similar to breathing exercises in *qigong*. Concentration is focused on a point just below the navel, that point being considered the center of *qi* (or *chi*, the life force, or life energy), and the point from which *qi* is believed to emanate throughout the body.

Students progress by learning a series of movements known collectively as a **form**. Students typically learn forms in class. Once the basics are mastered, forms can be practiced and perfected at home. Forms consist of twenty to one hundred moves practiced at a slow pace, requiring up to twenty minutes to complete.

The individual motions that comprise tai chi forms typically have descriptive, nature-based names, such as Wave Hands Like Clouds or Grasping the Bird's Tail

Alternative Spellings

Tai chi is also written as *t'ai chi, taijiquan, taiji,* and *t'ai-chi ch'uan.*

Concentration, careful attention to diaphragm breathing, and deliberate, slow motions characterize tai chi forms, which are based on observations of long-lived animals such as turtles and cranes.

(Figure 24). When students have attained proficiency, they may progress to "push hands," an exercise performed with a partner and designed to help students apply their knowledge of forms. In such exercises, students stand face to face, extending their arms and maintaining constant contact with their partners. Together they follow a prescribed series of movements, attempting to use their knowledge of the form while working with another person. Advanced practitioners may practice **free-form push hands**, in which a prescribed form is not used and each person attempts to upset his or her partner's balance without losing contact.

What Practitioners Say It Does

Adherents of Taoism and traditional Chinese medicine claim that the practice of tai chi, by strengthening and balancing a person's energy, can achieve both preventive and therapeutic effects. Balanced *qi* is believed to be central to health and well-being. Therefore, bringing about a balance of one's *qi* is said to ward off potential illness, improve general health, and extend life.

It is important to recall that tai chi rests on philosophical and spiritual ideas that remain essentially unchanged since their development thousands of years

Figure 24 Three of the ten positions that comprise the tai chi exercise Grasping the Bird's Tail.

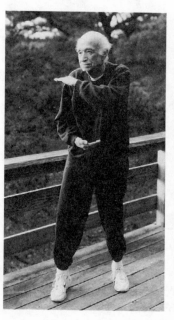
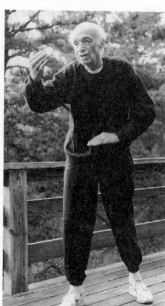
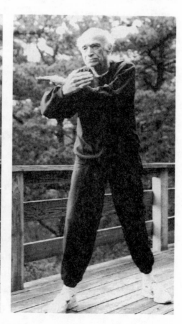

ago. Claims made for it stem from this historic background. Practitioners concede that some results claimed for this art, such as strengthening one's *qi* and improving harmony with the universe, are not easily quantified.

Documenting the core of this belief system—the existence of an invisible energy force called *qi*—remains an elusive goal. Other claims made for tai chi, however, are more readily observed and measured. These include its ability to enhance balance, strength, and flexibility. Documenting the effects of tai chi or showing that it works is one matter; proving the stated mechanisms of action, or how it works, is quite another.

Beliefs On Which It Is Based

Tai chi, *qigong*, and acupuncture are components of traditional Chinese medicine, which is based on the philosophy of Taoism. **Taoism** is a Chinese ideology initially expressed in the *Tao-Te Ching*, a book written in the sixth century B.C. Traditional Chinese medicine's most fundamental concepts include the existence of an invisible, internal energy or life force known as *qi*, and the idea of opposing forces and balances, which are usually expressed as yin and yang.

Yin and **Yang** refer to the balance of forces in the universe, an idea commonly represented by opposites such as male and female or light and dark. Tai chi movements are designed to express these forces in balanced and harmonious form. Movements are conducted in pairs of opposites. For example, a motion that ultimately involves turning to the right often begins with a slight move to the left. Initial moves often are designed to absorb the energy of the opponent's attack, while the second set of moves turns that energy back against the opponent.

Research Evidence to Date

Exercise generally is known to have healthful results. Tai chi in particular, however, was the subject of three major studies reported, respectively, in the *Journal of the American Medical Association* in 1995, the *Postgraduate Medical Journal* in 1996, and the *Journal of the American Geriatric Society* in 1996. The first publication described the results of a meta-analysis (a statistical analysis of many related studies) involving elderly people. It showed that tai chi and similar exercise programs improved physical balance and reduced the risk of falls.

The second publication, conducted by British researchers, compared three different cardiac rehabilitation programs (tai chi, aerobic exercise, and a nonexercise support group) for patients who had experienced heart attacks. At the end of eight weeks of practice, only tai chi had lowered the heart rate and blood pressure.

The third study involved 200 people over age seventy, showing that tai chi produces better stability than other balance-training techniques. The research found that elderly people can improve their balance and prevent falls by learning tai chi.

Just how tai chi accomplishes these goals—by balancing *qi* or by increasing aerobic strength and physical stability with practice as modern understanding would suggest—has yet to be scientifically determined.

What It Can Do for You

Tai chi exercises are said to result in qualities prized in Taoist philosophy: a soft and supple body produced by a strong and unblocked flow of *qi*; and harmony between body and mind enabled by the attainment of balance between yin and yang forces.

The measurement of *qi* eludes conventional science. Therefore, it is difficult to substantiate claims that tai chi can strengthen *qi* and bring about greater harmony with the universe. However, there are likely benefits to tai chi practice that do not rely on Taoist beliefs. Indeed, elderly Chinese can often be found in city parks in China in the early morning practicing tai chi movements and exhibiting ability and grace not often seen in Western people of similar age.

Like most moderate physical activities practiced on a regular basis, tai chi can improve all aspects of fitness, including stamina, agility, muscle tone, and flexibility. The practice of tai chi breathing exercises may serve a meditative function, thereby promoting stress reduction. Tai chi is particularly suited for older people and those who cannot practice difficult sports. Its movements are gentle, and it puts less stress on the body than

The Alternative Medicine Handbook

do other exercises or martial arts such as judo and karate.

Where to Get It

Tai chi is popular and available in most towns and cities. It is taught in health clubs, schools, YMCAs, community centers, and other facilities. Programs differ in their degree of emphasis on spiritual and fitness aspects of the art.

As with any exercise program, a good way to assess a teacher or an approach is to observe a class or participate in a trial class. Tai chi class fees are approximately $50 a month or less, although this depends on where you take the class.

Check your local library or bookstore for one of the many videotapes that augment classroom tai chi instruction. Type "tai chi" on your Internet searcher and find thousands of hits. Books are also available. An example is *The Complete Tai Chi: The Definitive Guide to Physical and Emotional Self Improvement,* by Master Alfred Huang (Charles E. Tuttle Co., Rutland, Vt. 1993).

41

Yoga

In Sanskrit, an ancient Indian language, *yoga* means "union," which captures its essence. Yoga is a disciplined activity, based on Hindu philosophy, that creates a union of mind, body, and spirit. It is a method by which one strives to experience the nature of reality, the divine spirit, or whatever phrase one assigns to a meaning greater than the self.

There are many branches and schools of yoga, each with a different route by which the higher state may be reached. **Hatha yoga**, which uses the body to achieve the goals of union and harmony, has captured the interest and devotion of many in the Western world. It is hatha yoga that we see on television and film, that is taught in most yoga classes, and that is marketed for its health and body-sculpting value in videotapes made by celebrities and fitness experts.

It aims to cultivate fitness, relaxation, and well-being, and can play a valuable role in stress reduction as a complementary therapy. Yoga's connections to ancient practices, Asian wisdom, and far-off lands are often part of its appeal.

What It Is

Hatha yoga is a 5,000-year-old set of exercises developed initially in India. Its three main components include proper breathing, movement, and posture. Yoga can be practiced in a group or individually. It involves completing a series of postures, such as standing on one leg while clasping the hands behind the head and holding the other leg out horizontally.

During the practice of postures, practitioners pay special attention to their breathing, exhaling while performing certain movements, and inhaling during others. Breathing is deep and from the diaphragm. Special breathing techniques are employed. In some yoga postures, for example, one inhales through a single nostril only, and exhales through the other nostril.

Special breathing is considered important for several reasons. Deep breathing promotes relaxation, and specific breathing rhythms assist in maintaining the postures. Also, yogic practice emphasizes the cultivation of *prana*, or life energy, and its practitioners believe that *prana* can be cultivated through breathing. *Prana* is similar to the *qi* of Chinese medicine, an invisible life force said to pervade human bodies and everything else in the universe.

A typical yoga class lasts from twenty minutes to an hour. The class begins with some warm-up poses and breathing exercises, and continues with a series of postures. Each posture is held for thirty seconds to several minutes. At the end of class, students may briefly practice meditation or lie down to rest for a brief time. There are different schools of hatha yoga in the West, which vary according to the intensity of their postures and whether the emphasis is placed on rigorous or gentle exercises.

Although postures achieved by advanced yoga students sometimes appear to defy anatomical limits, the purpose of hatha yoga is not contortion. Practice increases awareness of one's own body, and students learn both to know their own limitations and to move progressively toward more difficult postures (Figure 25).

What Practitioners Say It Does

Yoga was developed as part of a spiritual discipline. The purpose of yoga is to bring the practitioner to a higher state of awareness, an awareness of the divine nature and oneness of creation. By promoting disciplined focus on mind and body, yoga is said to enable a greater consciousness of daily life and of its divine origins.

Yoga as practiced in the West, however, tends to be used more as a method for physical and psychological change than for spiritual growth. Proponents of yoga as a means to the former believe that yoga can improve strength and flexibility and increase relaxation and well-being.

Beliefs on Which It Is Based

Yoga is closely related to the Hindu religion. Hatha yoga is part of the yogic tradition described by the yoga master Patanjali in his *Yoga Sutra* (probably written in the second century B.C.). It is thought to be the first attempt to compile the tradition and spiritual beliefs that

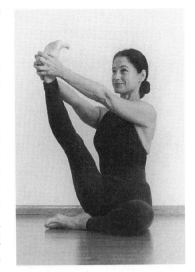

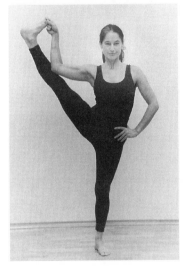

Figure 25 Not everyone can achieve this level of yoga excellence, but anyone can benefit from yoga exercises.

Reducing Pain and Stress through Bodywork

had been passed on verbally in previous millennia.

As practitioners move through the steps of Hatha yoga, they are said to move ever closer to the ultimate goal of realizing their divine natures. The steps are progressive, and students work to achieve increasingly greater control over body and mind. They work toward goals such as moral observance, self-discipline, concentration, and meditation. Hatha yoga focuses on the breath control and posture. It was developed because, according to Hindu belief, we continue, as we have since prehistory, to live in a dark age of spiritual decline, and hatha yoga is necessary to elevate the body and mind.

Research Evidence to Date

A substantial amount of research has been conducted on the effects of yoga. Research shows that yoga practice can induce physiological change, increase skin resistance (a measure of reduced stress), cause the heart to work more efficiently, decrease respiratory rate and blood pressure, improve physical fitness, and produce brain-wave activity indicative of relaxation. Based on this body of evidence, yoga has been incorporated into complementary treatment regimens for many illnesses. It is also used independently as a fitness exercise and as a method of stress reduction.

Yoga has been used as complementary therapy for heart disease, asthma, diabetes, drug addiction, HIV/AIDS, migraine headaches, cancer, and arthritis to reduce stress and increase flexibility and strength. California cardiologist Dean Ornish includes yoga in his diet and exercise-based heart disease reversal program. With severe dietary modifications and other relaxation techniques, many stress reduction programs use yoga to achieve their goals. Yoga techniques are documented to reduce stress and anxiety not only immediately following the activity, but also for lasting periods of time.

What It Can Do for You

People who practice yoga on a regular basis typically experience lowered levels of stress and increased feelings of relaxation and well-being. Yoga enhances physical fitness, and it helps relieve symptoms of chronic illness such as anxiety and pain.

The Alternative Medicine Handbook

In practicing yoga for its health benefits, three caveats should be observed:

1. Yoga is a complementary therapy, not a cure for disease. Although it improves patients' feelings of well-being and enhances quality of life, the practice of yoga does not diminish illnesses or the need for ongoing medical treatment.

2. Yoga requires regular practice to be effective. Many people do not have the time for this commitment, which may require several hours weekly at a minimum.

3. The nature of some of the postures can be stressful to people with particular health problems. Therefore, as with beginning any exercise program, people under medical care should consult their physicians to be sure yoga is appropriate.

Where to Get It

There are many books, videos, magazines and on-line media resources devoted to yoga:

✦ One book considered a classic is *The Complete Illustrated Book of Yoga*, by Swami Vishnudevananda (Harmony Books, New York, 1980).

✦ Many yoga schools, individuals with interests in yoga, and yoga teachers have established home pages on the World Wide Web. These home pages often contain explanations of various aspects of yoga.

✦ The *Yoga Journal* magazine, 2054 University Avenue, Berkeley, CA 94704 (510 841-9200) is available at health-food stores and some bookstores. It offers a directory of close to one thousand yoga teachers in its July/August issue every year.

A good teacher can help the beginner a great deal. Classes are offered by many public schools, YMCAs, recreation centers, community centers, and schools dedicated specifically to yoga. When you locate a yoga teacher in your area, observe students in action or take an introductory class. Talk to students who have studied with that teacher for some time. Ask the teacher how long he or she has studied and taught yoga. Become informed and feel comfortable with that particular class before you sign up.

PART SIX

ENHANCING WELL-BEING THROUGH THE SENSES

We have all experienced the satisfaction of drawing or painting, playing or listening to a favorite piece of music, telling or hearing a good joke or a funny story. These impulses toward creativity and joy may be used not just for aesthetic satisfaction, but also for healing. That is what the practitioners and clients of the therapies described in this part believe.

Most of these therapies share several broad concepts and purposes. They appeal to and engage one or more of the senses; they involve creating or experiencing a work of art; and they require that patients take an active role in their own care. The application of sound and light may require less from the patient and may be less artistically expressive, but advocates of these regimens also claim clinical benefits.

It is important here as with other types of treatments to separate therapies that claim to cure disease (alternative therapies) from those used as adjuncts to mainstream medical treatment or to enhance well-being (complementary therapies). Most of the methods in this part are used appropriately as complementary techniques. They can decrease anxiety, promote relaxation, and create distraction for patients with major illness such as cancer, AIDS, and Alzheimer's disease.

However, almost every therapy in this part, as well as those elsewhere in the book, has a few fringe advocates who claim miracle cures. A few advocates of light therapy, for example, promote it as a cure for cancer, a promise as dangerous as it is untrue.

Despite some unproven claims for light and sound therapies, both light and sound are used in conventional medicine. Light therapy successfully treats seasonal affective disorder (SAD), a psychiatric syndrome of depression caused by reduced natural light in winter months. Sound is used in conventional medicine for both diagnosis and treatment in the form of **ultrasound**, or high-frequency (outside of human hearing range) sound waves. Ultrasound used for diagnostic purposes explores the heart, checks fetal development, and examines other areas of the body, painlessly and easily. In one treatment, ultrasonic waves are sent through water to painlessly enter the body and destroy kidney stones.

Therapies that use the senses typically are inexpensive and free of side effects. They can be practiced easily alone or with others, with or without a professional therapist, on an outpatient basis or by patients who are hospitalized.

Most of the therapies in this part are relatively new, having been organized less than a few decades ago. Music therapy formally began in the 1950s, and a professional organization for dance therapy was established only in 1966. At the same time, most of these approaches spring from roots that extend back to the beginning of civilization. Visual arts, dance, humor, aromatherapy, chanting, and music have been intrinsic components of human culture for thousands of years.

Practitioners of these therapies often began as performers or students of the art, and then became interested in its medical applications. Dance therapy emerged when modern dance instructors saw the positive results of dance on their students and perceived its healing potential. The fine art therapies share the common belief that creativity is inherently therapeutic.

Art, music, and dance therapists are facilitators. They provide patients with the tools, advice, and emotional support that enable them to use their creative energies. Some effects are emotional, others help the body, and a few accomplish both. Because these activities involve listening to music, producing

The Alternative Medicine Handbook

art, dancing, and creating and responding to humor, they seem more like prescriptions for a balanced existence rather than medical interventions—as indeed they are. These fulfilling activities also are part of wellness programs that include maintaining good nutrition, exercise, and healthy relationships.

These primarily noninvasive therapies aim to engage the senses. Such activities are pleasant and rewarding, but they may also distract or focus attention away from the emotional and physical pain of illness. Finally, these therapies are active; they help patients interact with their environment through their perceptions and reactions to the world. Most require that patients do something, rather than have something done for or to them, as is more typical during illness. These therapies often can induce a sense of control that is lacking during serious illness. Enabling a child or adult with cancer to draw gives that person an active means of expression, a tool with which fears and feelings about their disease can be communicated.

A few scientific studies have evaluated the merits of therapies involving the senses. Research indicates that certain sounds and aromas can promote relaxation, and that listening to Mozart can enhance some mental tasks. The therapies in this chapter do not cure disease. There is evidence, however, that they produce physiological as well as psychological benefits. They can increase wellness and quality of life regardless of one's health status.

42 ∼
Aromatherapy

A combination of folk wisdom and accident merged to become the modern practice of aromatherapy. Aromatherapy involves the use of oils distilled from plants for therapeutic purposes. It has a long history of use in ancient Egypt, China, and India. The distillation method used to extract essential oils was invented by an Arab physician in the tenth century A.D.

Modern aromatherapy in the West began with a French chemist, René Gattefosse. Working one day in the laboratory at his family's perfume company, he burned his hand. He quickly doused his hand with some readily available lavender oil. The burn healed quickly and left no scar, perking his interest in the possible curative effects of plant oils. He began to study them, coining the term *aromatherapy* in the 1930s to describe this new field.

What It Is

Aromatherapy is the use of **essential oils**, which are natural, high-quality, pure oils derived from the distillation of plants. The oils are named for the plant from which they are derived, such as lavender, rose, eucalyptus. They are highly concentrated: between fifty and several thousand pounds of plant material is required to make one pound of essential oil, depending on the plant. At least forty essential oils are used in aromatherapy. Each is categorized according to its effects on the body, mind, and diseases it is said to treat. Oils from various plants may be used individually or in combinations.

Aromatherapy is delivered to patients in several ways. Oils can be applied directly to the skin through massage or as a liniment. For skin application, the oils are combined with a carrier medium, usually a vegetable oil, because the amount of essential oil required is so small.

The oils also may be inhaled with steaming water containing a few drops of an essence, or by using diffusers to spread steam containing an oil throughout a room. Because they are highly concentrated and therefore potentially toxic, the oils should not be taken internally.

Aromatherapy can be self-administered or received

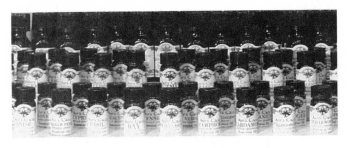

Figure 26 Aromatherapy oils can make a warm bath even more pleasant.

from a practitioner. Several organizations in Europe and North America train and certify aromatherapists. Aromatherapists sometimes combine knowledge of aromatherapy with other forms of alternative practice, such as traditional Chinese healing or herbal medicine.

What Practitioners Say It Does

Aromatherapy has three main functions. The first is stress reduction, which is achieved primarily through the personal use of aromatic oils in one's workplace or home, or by combining aromatherapy with other stress reduction activities, such as soaking in a hot bath treated with scented oil or receiving a massage accompanied by aromatherapy.

The second function is preventive. According to some advocates, aromatherapy can balance and increase the well-being of both body and mind, thus decreasing the likelihood that disease will develop. The third function is therapeutic. Aromatherapy is used to treat physical and mental ailments. Lavender, for example, is used to treat anxiety, mild depression, and insomnia.

Some Popular Aromatherapies and Results Claimed for Them

Plant	Effects Claimed
Lemon	Detoxifies; stimulates immune system and liver
Vetivert	Regulates hormones, stimulates glands and nervous system
Rosemary	Relieves pain; relaxes muscles
Peppermint	Provides pain and digestive relief; decreases inflammation
Camomile	Serves as sedative, relaxant, and antiallergen
Eucalyptus	Eliminates infection
Rose	Regulates female hormones
Lavender	Calms, sedates, relaxes; lowers blood pressure

Enhancing Well-Being through the Senses

Conditions that practitioners believe to be aided by aromatherapy include acne, anxiety, cold and flu, skin disorders, headaches, indigestion, premenstrual syndrome, muscle tension, and pain. Some aromatherapy advocates use body applications (massages and liniments) to treat physical problems, and inhalation methods to treat emotional problems.

Beliefs on Which It Is Based

Aromatherapy rests on two central principles, one well known to conventional science and the other as yet unproven. The first is that aromatherapy is based on the sense of smell, which is extremely acute in humans and other animals. Very small amounts of a scent trigger the sense of smell by activating receptors in the nasal cavity. These receptors are neurons, or nerve cells, which translate the odor into nerve impulses, enabling them to travel instantly to the olfactory bulb, which is part of the limbic system, the area of the brain that scientists have identified with memory and emotion. The sense of smell has been studied extensively for its role in communication and memory.

The second, but unproven, belief on which aromatherapy is based is that essential oils, through the sense of smell or by absorption through the skin, can affect the body's health.

Research Evidence to Date

Substantial research evidence exists about the olfactory system (the sense of smell). For example, a single waft of an odor can trigger memories from decades back. This was captured in Marcel Proust's famous passage in his novel, *Remembrance of Things Past*, when the author was flooded with childhood memories as he bit into a *madeleine*, a French tea cake made for him as a child.

In addition, scientists have found substances called **pheromones** in almost all organisms. These chemicals are emitted by the body and sensed by the olfactory system. In mammals, pheromones play a role in sexual attraction and mating. In other organisms, they facilitate not only mating, but also the attraction of prey and forms of communication. Pheromones are responsible for a phenomenon called menstrual synchrony, where the menstrual cycles of women who live in close proximity often become similar, or synchronize with one another.

Some studies implicate the sense of smell in illness and relaxation. One researcher found that certain odors could trigger migraines in some individuals and, alternatively, that the fragrance of green apples may heighten feelings of relaxation.

However, although smell and the olfactory system have multiple functions, there is no scientific evidence—no controlled studies—indicating that aromatherapy can aid in preventing or alleviating disease. The medical literature contains no research on the effects of aromatherapy as a medical treatment.

What It Can Do for You

Like other complementary methods, aromatherapy may reduce stress, enhance pleasure, and improve quality of life for those to whom it appeals. However, no evidence in the medical literature supports claims by proponents that aromatherapy can help prevent or heal disease. Evidence is lacking even in the case of those minor and self-limiting conditions, such as headaches and colds, that advocates say can be alleviated or abbreviated by aromatherapy.

Used as a strictly complementary technique, however, aromatherapy is a pleasant addition to baths and massages (Figure 26). Scented candles or aroma sprays, for those who enjoy the fragrance, contribute to a sense of relaxation and help create a calming atmosphere.

Where to Get It

There are several popular books on aromatherapy if you want to try it on your own. *Aromatherapy for Common Ailments*, by Shirley Price (Simon and Schuster, New York, 1991), is but one example.

Organizations of aromatherapists can help you locate sources of essential oils and aromatherapists in your area. Trade organizations for aromatherapy include:

✦ American Alliance of Aromatherapy
  P.O. Box 750428
  Petaluma, CA 94975-0428
  Telephone: (707) 778-6762

A Few Caveats

The essential oils of aromatherapy never should be ingested by mouth or taken into the body through other routes.

Also, prolonged, extensive exposure to essential oils should be avoided, as reports in the medical literature indicate that such use has produced allergic reactions in some people.

- American Aromatherapy Association
  P.O. Box 3679
  South Pasadena, CA 91031
  Telephone: (818) 457-1742
- National Association of Holistic Aromatherapy
  P.O. Box 17622
  Boulder, CO 80308-0622
  Telephone: (303) 258-3791

43 Art Therapy

Art that results from the creative process is an end in and of itself. Art therapy, by contrast, is a means to an end. It uses creative activity as a vehicle for rehabilitation, a means of helping the sick or disabled.

Art therapists believe that everyone is an artist, or can be when left to create freely and without external constraints of judgment or criticism. The very process of creating a painting, sculpture, or any other type of art helps develop self-awareness and self-esteem. The release of creative energy generates internal activity that helps produce physical, mental, and spiritual healing. For those who cannot themselves create, the opportunity to experience the art of others can produce similar benefits.

Many people, including patients under treatment for physical or emotional illnesses, have difficulty verbalizing their fears. The resulting repressed feelings exacerbate tension and unease. Visual art, followed perhaps by pondering its apparent and symbolic meaning, can be cathartic and rewarding.

What It Is

Visual art therapy is based on the belief that the creative process is intrinsically therapeutic. Therapists provide relevant equipment and tools, technical advice, and emotional support. Patients are free to draw, paint, sculpt, or involve themselves in other forms of visual artistic expression or appreciation as they prefer and are able. Art therapy can occur in people's homes, in art studios, or in hospital beds. It is used as a means of expressing sometimes hidden emotions, and to gain benefits provided by the act of creation.

What Practitioners Say It Does

Some art therapists view the act of creating as the primary goal. In particular circumstances, however, creativity may be less important than insight or expressing feelings. Images are mental constructs, personal messages sent by individuals to themselves. The expression of those images through art offers an opportunity to contact oneself through the senses, and to create a tangible record of sensations, perceptions, and feelings.

Art therapy is said to support self-esteem, foster development of a sense of identity, and promote healing through the maturation of creativity. Feelings expressed by patients' interactions with various media can be translated into words more readily than feelings kept inside can.

In addition to helping the patient, art therapy can also be helpful to those working with the patients. The visual images the patient creates provide a tangible, permanent record of the patient's state of mind at that time and allow the therapist, artist, nurse, or educator to access the patient's emotions. Art therapy can create order out of chaos by giving form to images and emotions, and it encourages a silent dialogue between the patient's inner sensations and external realities. Viewing or producing paintings, drawings, and other forms of art can help keep patients from remaining passive recipients during treatment for chronic or psychiatric diseases.

Beliefs on Which It Is Based

Art therapy is based on the belief that the act of creating or viewing a visible product enables patients to express and communicate inner emotions, which is thought to be helpful to the healing process.

Research shows that infants, children, and adults during times of severe stress or threat of life typically encode memory visually and through sensory channels, bypassing the conscious or verbal memory systems. Art therapy allows such nonverbal memories and feelings to surface so that they can be confronted and hopefully managed.

Another belief on which art therapy is based is that the beauty of creative works is intrinsically uplifting and refreshing. The timeless nature of great works of art that continue to elicit powerful feelings from people all over the world in all walks of life is testament to the power of art. Part of that power is distraction, the ability of art as we view it to remove us mentally from the constraints and problems of our physical or emotional pain. This, too, can contribute to healing by reducing stress and enhancing well-being.

Many Benefits

The act of expression as well as the ability to view works of art appears to have many strongly felt, albeit undocumented, benefits.

Research Evidence to Date

The medical literature contains very little about art therapy. The few articles that have been published consist of descriptive reports rather than research studies. They describe art therapy programs, staff assessments, and therapists' perceptions of patient improvement. Positive reports exist for psychiatric patients, people with spinal cord injury, those suffering chronic stress and serious illness, disabled people in rehabilitation programs, and Alzheimer's patients.

The paucity of research belies the extensive amount of activity in this area. Many medical centers and some cancer centers hold art exhibits of patients' work, and such work has been published in full-color catalogs by several institutions. The walls of some hospitals display professional works of art. Often, these are rotating exhibits donated by local artists or galleries. Professional artists conduct workshops to teach patients, families, and hospital staff how to use art as therapy.

Projects and activities of this kind are believed to foster physical, mental, and spiritual healing, and to contribute to the well-being not only of patients but their caregivers and families as well. They are thought to enhance self-awareness, self-esteem, and creative energy and to improve mood and reduce feelings of distress, loneliness, and anxiety.

What It Can Do for You

Art therapy allows patients to express hidden emotions, a process that may encourage or assist the healing process. Art therapy does not cure disease; it is a supplement to medical practice and a complementary therapy. Some patients can manage only a passive form of art therapy involving viewing displays of art. Other patients may actively create. Either way, art therapy appears to improve well-being, enhance quality of life, and provide distractions during times of difficulty. Creative energy—one's own or another's—may assist healing and help patients cope with or overcome physical and mental distress (Figure 27).

Where to Get It

Your hospital or other inpatient facility may have

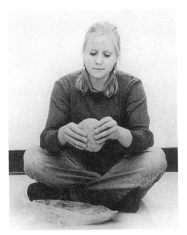

Figure 27 Sculpting is both an art and an art therapy.

someone on staff who could arrange an art program, or you can contact the national association:

+ American Art Therapy Association
  1202 Allanson Road
  Mundelein, IL 60060
  Telephone: (708) 949-6064

⌒44
Dance
Therapy

The use of dance as a therapeutic tool may be as old as dance itself. For early humankind, dance was an outlet for expression, a means of communicating feelings, and a way to commune with nature. Dance rituals usually accompanied rites of passage, ceremonies by which individuals were admitted into adulthood or integrated into the community. In the earliest civilizations, dance was part of that entwined combination of religion, medicine, and magic. The ritual dance of the priest or shaman (medicine man), was central to the oldest forms of communal activity. Dance also provided a socially accepted means of releasing tension and improving physical and mental well-being.

The great anthropologist Sir James George Frazer had a tremendous impact on the modern dance movement. In his book *The Golden Bough: A Study in Magic and Religion* (1890), he examined the role of ritual dance in primitive cultures. His insights provided new information about the anthropological importance of dance that broadened understanding of its meaning and value, and this led eventually to the emergence of dance therapy. The original purposes of dance—expressing magic, religion, and spirituality—were revived and integrated into modern dance and, shortly thereafter, into dance therapy.

The roots of dance therapy extend back to the early 1900s. Most major dance therapy pioneers began their careers as accomplished modern dancers. Their broad experience in teaching and performing led naturally to an appreciation for the therapeutic potential of dance. The modern dance movement was a reaction to the social and intellectual climate of the time, a rebellion against established forms of art, and part of the broader effort to liberate the individual from societal constraints.

What It Is

Dance therapy is the use of dance movement to assist healing or enhance well-being. For decades, dance therapy was viewed as the province of individuals with unique skills rather than as a profession. Dance therapy

took its first steps toward professional recognition and
respect in 1966 when the American Dance Therapy
Association (ADTA) was established.

A formal definition of dance therapy was developed
and revised in 1972 to read: "Dance therapy is the psy-
chotherapeutic use of movement as a process which fur-
thers the emotional and physical integration of the individual."

What Practitioners Say It Does

Dance therapists believe that their work assists
patients in every aspect of their selves. On an emotional level, dance therapy is used to promote body image
and encourage self-expression. It may also assist in
explorating and resolving emotional issues such as
anger, frustration, and loss.

Intellectual improvement is another goal of dance
therapy. Levels of awareness appear to sharpen for
some patients, and cognition, motivation, and memory
may improve.

Dance therapy also can assist physical coordination
and motor skills. The use of repetition and the rhythm of
the music provide a structure that helps people organize
movement and, at the same time, clarify thought processes. Both enhance functional and recreational skills.

The abilities to socialize and communicate are
improved with dance therapy. The self-expression that
dance requires increases the individual's self-confidence
and self-awareness. Dance therapy has even helped
severely disturbed psychiatric patients, sometimes
assisting them to communicate for the first time.

Dance therapy has been tried with the physically
handicapped. Self-confidence and well-being can be promoted while expanding the individual's perception of
movement. In the last decade, dance therapists have
branched into many new areas, expanding therapeutic
dance to reach new communities. These include trou-
bled families, people with eating disorders, sexually
abused children, and patients with traumatic brain
injuries.

Beliefs on Which It Is Based

Advocates believe that the body and mind are inseparable, and that body movement reflects our inner emotional states. Physical motion provides the benefits of exercise, and it is believed also to encourage positive thoughts and emotions that will help promote health and growth.

Dance therapy is based on the belief that people can regain a sense of completeness by experiencing a unity of body, mind, and spirit through dance.

Research Evidence to Date

The medical literature contains articles on the benefits of dance therapy with adolescent and adult psychiatric patients, the elderly, children with learning disabilities, deaf people, mentally handicapped children and adults, and people in nursing homes.

Dance therapy with the elderly was one of the earliest efforts. Problems common to the elderly typically include physical limitations, dependency on others, social isolation, loneliness, loss of self-esteem, death of peers, and fear of one's own death. These problems add stress to individuals who may have few if any outlets for releasing tension.

Dance therapy can provide such an outlet. It emphasizes interpersonal interaction, sharing, and support, and it addresses the individual's need for physical exercise and expression. The psychological focus strives to encourage the expression of emotions and to enhance feelings of self-worth and well-being (Figure 28).

Blind or visually impaired patients have a hard time at

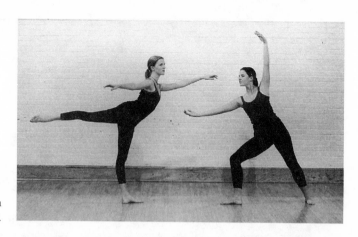

Figure 28 Dancing can make your spirits soar.

first with dance therapy, because they tend to be frightened of moving. Once they feel safe and believe they are in a secure environment, they become willing to explore creative movement, eventually increasing their range, scope, and depth of motion in dance. Dance therapy also is effective with individuals who are partially or totally deaf.

What It Can Do for You

The dance experience for disabled individuals helps reduce feelings of isolation, and motivates social relationships in a group setting. This is especially important for deaf and blind individuals, because they can withdraw and become socially isolated if they find communication too difficult to pursue. Physical education or physical therapy often is not available for them, and their muscular capacity may deteriorate as a result. This problem is due to the social isolation that can occur, not to any inherent physical weakness. Dance movement as part of physical education can enhance muscle strength and coordination for the disabled as well as for others.

Dance therapy provides the opportunity to express feelings and release tension by moving freely. It can be relaxing, exhilarating, empowering—an act of creative expression with important personal rewards regardless of physical or emotional abilities or limitations.

Where to Get It

For information and advice, contact:
✦ American Dance Therapy Association

2000 Century Plaza, Suite 108
Columbia, MD 21044
Telephone: (410) 997-4040
✦ Laban/Bartenieff Institute of Movement Studies
11 East Fourth Street, Third Floor
New York, NY 10003
Telephone: (212) 477-4299

45

Humor Therapy

On his return flight home from a trip to Moscow in the mid-1960s, Norman Cousins, then editor of the *Saturday Review*, became rapidly ill. Within two days of landing in the United States, he was hospitalized with high fever, severe pain, and difficulty moving his arms and legs. After two weeks of hospitalization, his condition slowly worsened while his physicians struggled to treat a debilitating problem that eluded specific diagnosis.

In a now famous story, Cousins checked himself out of the hospital and into a nearby hotel. He began a self-invented regimen of laughter and massive doses of vitamin C. A film projector was brought to the hotel room, and each day Mr. Cousins watched Marx Brothers films and episodes of *Candid Camera*. These were his favorite comedy routines, and they elicited continual laughter despite the pain.

In fact, the pain began to decrease as the sessions of laughter continued. The illness relented, eventually disappearing entirely. It never recurred. Cousins' doctors could not explain his recovery in medical terms. Cousins later published an article in the *New England Journal of Medicine* and popularized this experience in a book, *Anatomy of an Illness*. His works set off a wave of interest in the potential therapeutic benefits of laughter and humor. Cousins himself was appointed as a faculty member of the Medical School dean's office at the University of California, Los Angeles, where he worked on mind-body issues.

Although Cousins's recovery cannot be attributed with any certainty to the humor and laughter he experienced, laughter may well have contributed to it. Furthermore, it no doubt enhanced the quality of his life, as it does for a wide variety of patients.

What It Is

Humor or laughter therapy is the deliberate use of humor as a complementary treatment for people suffering from physical or emotional disorders. In medical facilities, laughter therapy may be available in a special room in the hospital or ambulatory care facility. These are rooms where patients can go to relax and get away temporarily from the institutional environment. Typically, they contain small libraries that include humorous books, videos, toys, and other amusing objects.

Some hospitals have volunteers who wheel carts filled with books, toys, audio and videotapes, and other objects to patients' rooms. Trained laughter therapists are available in some towns, and patients or family members often try humor therapy on their own.

A hospital in Charlotte, North Carolina, set up a "Laughmobile" containing video and audiotapes, Play-Doh, coloring books, puzzles, and games. It was used with great success for adults and children hospitalized for cancer treatment. In other states, volunteers have established transportable humor and laughter programs, consisting of cartons of materials that they bring to inpatient facilities when invited. The materials include, among other items, rubber chickens and water pistols, which patients apparently use to everyone's amusement with their physicians and dietary staff.

Humor also involves one-on-one interactions between patients and caregivers. Of course, anyone can follow Norman Cousins's example of reading, listening to, or viewing what they find funny. Because people differ in what makes them laugh, laughter therapy is individualized.

What Practitioners Say It Does

Laughter as a complementary therapy is recognized as helpful for many patient groups in many medical circumstances, all of which are complementary. Advocates do not claim that humor or laughter cures disease.

Humor therapy is brought to cancer patients, sick children, people under treatment for depression, the elderly in nursing homes, cardiac patients, and other groups. The therapeutic goal is to improve quality of life, provide symptom relief by distracting the patient from constant awareness of pain, and improve emotional and psychological health by encouraging relaxation and stress reduction. As part of support programs for patients, humor can provide a means of communication between patients and their caregivers and loved ones.

According to Proverbs 17:22, "a merry heart doeth good like a medicine," and an old Irish saying terms "a good laugh and a long sleep the best cures in the doctor's book."

Often it does this by serving as an icebreaker, allowing patients to convey ideas or feelings that are difficult or awkward to express in other ways.

Beliefs on Which It Is Based

Although common sense would seem to be the rationale for including laughter and humor in patient care settings, laughter has a long history in medical practice. Laughter was used as an "anesthetic" to distract patients during surgical procedures in the thirteenth century, and other references to it appear in ancient medical literature. Accounts of the physiological benefits of laughter are also found in the American medical literature from the early years of the twentieth century.

The physiological effects of laughter include an increase in heart rate, breathing rate, and oxygen consumption, which in turn stimulate the circulatory system. Laughter also massages and exercises the muscles and organs involved in breathing, as well as causing the release of endorphins, which are the body's natural morphinelike compounds that help control pain. These physiological effects, advocates believe, explain the therapeutic benefits of laughter and humor (Figure 29).

Research Evidence to Date

There are no scientific studies comparing the effects of laughter on people who receive humor as a complementary therapy versus those who do not. However,

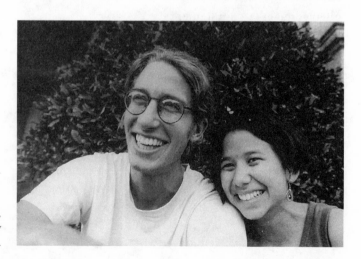

Figure 29 Laughter is, indeed, good medicine with many therapeutic benefits.

The Alternative Medicine Handbook

research has documented the physiological effects of laughter, and anecdotal reports describe patients' appreciation and positive experiences with humor and laughter.

Recent university-based research found that laughing lowers blood pressure and increases muscle flexibility in addition to releasing endorphins. **Endorphins** not only reduce pain; they also induce a degree of euphoria, and therefore may further enhance the positive effects of laughter.

Furthermore, there is some preliminary evidence indicating that laughter increases immune activity, and that it can reduce levels of cortisol, a stress hormone associated with suppressing the immune system. The results of other investigations show that laughter increases natural killer cell activity in the immune system. These studies are preliminary, and so far have limited clinical implications.

What It Can Do for You

Laughter and humor are distracting and uplifting. Humor helps people cope with stress and illness, and it creates an environment that is relaxing. Being with friends with whom one can laugh easily seems to enhance quality of life for people generally.

Despite its clear virtues, humor is not a replacement for conventional medical treatment. Even Norman Cousins, whose diagnosis and cure were uncertain, cautioned in his writings and in later work at the UCLA Medical School against trying to use humor instead of medical treatment for illness.

Where to Get It

If you are hospitalized, ask what facilities or programs exist for relaxation and humor. You may ask the hospital or visitors for video- or audiotapes, or ask visitors to bring you humorous books. Beyond that, life itself is a good source of humor. Humor is an individual response, and what sends you into gales of laughter may leave another blank-eyed and unmoved. Yet humor is one of the easiest therapies to incorporate in your life, whether you are ill or well.

46 ⬿

Light Therapy

All living things respond to daily and seasonal cycles of light and dark. **Circadian rhythm**, also called the body's inner clock, is the term applied to the regular repetition of light cycles in humans and other living organisms. **Chronobiology** is the scientific study of the cyclic effects of time on living systems.

There are numerous and varied examples of how light influences the behavior of plants and animals. Some flowers open wide at first light in the morning and close their petals at night. World travelers suffer from jet lag, which is due at least in part to the interruption of habitual day-night light cycles. Depression is more prevalent among people in northern latitudes where daylight in winter months is substantially shortened or nonexistent. Similarly, depression in North America is more common during winter months when there are fewer hours of sunlight. Bright white light, much more intense than typical workplace lighting, is used in some offices and factories to increase work efficiency and reduce drowsiness, particularly for night-shift workers.

Cycles of night and day, or darkness and light, can change body temperature, vary hormone production, and alter the length of time that people sleep. This occurs because light enters the body through the eyes and is transmitted as electrical impulses along the optic nerve to the brain, where it affects the body's physiological functions and health.

The effects of light are not uniformly positive. Ultraviolet (UV) light from the sun, for example, is a primary cause of skin cancer, yet the full spectrum of light emanating from the sun, taken in moderation, is healthful and a major source of vitamin D.

What It Is

Light therapy, in the form of **light boxes** that shine bright light into the room during darker winter days, is used by psychiatrists to treat **seasonal affective disorder** (SAD), a type of depression that occurs during seasons when days have many dark and few sunlit hours. Research substantiates the ability of this treatment to reduce depression. (Light boxes prescribed to treat depression should not be confused with tanning booths. The latter are dangerous because they can cause skin cancer and premature wrinkling due to the release of large amounts of UV radiation, whereas light boxes have too little UV radiation to produce a tan.) Light boxes for SAD are not considered alternative medicine; they represent an accepted, proven mainstream treatment.

Many claims are made for light therapy as an alternative healing method for conditions other than SAD. In alternative light therapy, various types of light from different sources are prescribed inappropriately to treat many diagnoses. Types of light include full-spectrum or natural sunlight, bright-light therapy, UV light, colored-light therapy, and various laser therapies. Advocates claim effectiveness in treating a wide range of maladies including bulimia, psoriasis, symptoms of AIDS, and even breast, rectal, and colon cancers. These claims are not proven; in many cases they do not even appear logical. Light therapy should never be used instead of mainstream treatment for these or any other medical illness. Some of these therapies are described below.

UV light therapy applies different wavelengths of ultraviolet light, identified as UV-A, UV-B, and UV-C. The UV-B wavelength is the most damaging to skin. These and other types of light are used as alternatives to mainstream care to "treat" autoimmune disorders, to attack bacteria and body toxins, and to treat pigmentation problems and other disorders.

Colored-light therapy using red, blue, violet, white, and occasionally other colors, sometimes with flashing patterns, are used to treat sleep disorders, shoulder pain, diabetes, impotence, allergies, and many other symptoms.

Photodynamic therapy is a variation of colored-light therapy. Dyes injected directly into skin cancer tumors are claimed to absorb different colors of light and kill the cancer cells. A process called "syntonic optometry" (a process not found in standard medical dictionaries or texts) directs colored lights into the eyes to "influence" brain functions.

What Practitioners Say It Does

The traditional and accepted benefits of light include

serving as a source of vitamin D, optimizing working conditions, and maintaining the normal circadian rhythm function with all of its benefits. Preliminary evidence suggests that natural light may be effective in treating jaundice in newborns.

Great care must be taken in responding to other claims for light therapy. Claims include promises that light therapy will cure or promote the healing of several types of cancer; reduce hyperactivity in school children; relieve headaches and other ailments; and help regulate sexual function, the immune system, breathing, and digestion. These claims are not substantiated by clinical research.

Beliefs on Which It Is Based

Practitioners of alternative light therapy propound beliefs far beyond known facts. A California osteopathic physician, for example, states that visually perceived light can affect the parts of the brain that control learning, memory, and motor skills, thereby enhancing these capacities. Too much artificial light without enough natural light, another advocate states, interferes with the body's ability to absorb nutrients, a condition that advocates term "malillumination." An acupuncturist in California combines cold lasers with acupuncture in the belief that this helps wound healing and balances energy flow in the acupuncture meridians that are said to traverse the length of the body (see Chapter 1).

A system labeled **chromatotherapy** is based on a belief that shining colored lights on the body will have a beneficial effect on cancer. Proponents hold that red light benefits the blood, yellow light the liver, and so on.

Other, similar approaches exist, claiming that various colors of light will cure all diseases. They do not.

Research Evidence to Date

There is no scientific research on alternative light therapies. The medical literature during the past ten years contains one article that mentions it. However, it refers to light therapy only to discredit a popular alternative medicine book that claims light therapy can cure breast cancer.

What It Can Do for You

Proper amounts of exposure to sunlight can contribute to one's good health by promoting a consistent circadian rhythm and exposure to vitamin D, which is required for maintaining healthy teeth and bones and for absorbing calcium. Working in adequately lighted workspaces usually reduces eyestrain and fatigue, and promotes more normal sleep habits. Adding artificial light in the form of light boxes helps reduce the depression that often accompanies inadequate exposure to natural sunlight. Light boxes may also help treat jaundice in infants and some skin conditions.

It is what light therapy cannot do for you that must be carefully examined. There is no acceptable evidence that light therapy in any of its manifestations will cure cancer, arthritis, menstrual difficulties, tooth decay, hair loss, Alzheimer's disease, or any of the remaining diseases and conditions it promises to dispel.

Where to Get It

+ For information on full-spectrum lighting, contact the Environmental Health and Light Institute in Tampa, Florida (800 544-4878).
+ The Society for Light Treatment and Biological Rhythms has an office in Wilsonville, Oregon (503 694-2404).
+ At least four books on light and color therapy have been published since 1988. Buyer beware.

47

Music Therapy

Listen to a few bars of a song on the radio, and our immediate surroundings melt away, the melody carrying us back to where we heard it first. We link music to the milestones of life, both joyous and sorrowful. Sports arenas blast pounding rock music to arouse crowds. Colleges have "fight songs" for the same end.

Business offices, factories, and retail stores long ago learned the value of piped-in music to provide more beneficial environments in which to work or sell more goods. In fact, the idea of background or "elevator music" as a benefit to business created an entire new industry, developed by the Muzak system and marketed throughout commerce and industry.

We have all experienced the pleasing sounds of music that can lull us to sleep, develop a romantic mood, or stir us to tap in time to the beat. Music is used in hospital birthing rooms, newborn nurseries, and operating suites to promote the desired effect on patients and staff. Can the undeniable power of music to arouse our emotions and change our mood be used in medicine?

What It Is

Music therapy is the use of music to encourage healing and promote a general sense of well-being. Patients listen to or perform music under the guidance of a professionally trained and certified music therapist. Music therapists perform, listen to music with patients, analyze their lyrics, write songs, and join in music improvisation. Patients can play or listen to music, based on their previous experience and current condition (Figure 30). After assessing a patient's condition, the music therapist selects the type of music therapy most appropriate for that particular patient.

Sometimes music therapy is conducted on a group basis, where patients listen to or play music with groups of friends and loved ones or with other patients with the same condition. The music therapist may select music with the patient's active input, finding songs and melodies that have special meaning or ability to relax that individual.

From The Art of Preserving Health, Book IV, by John Armstrong, 1709-1779:

"Music exalts each Joy, allays each Grief, expels Diseases, softens every Pain, subdues the rage of Poison and the Plague."

The Alternative Medicine Handbook

The formal discipline of music therapy in the United States can be traced back to the granting of degrees in music therapy in the late 1940s and the use of music therapy with disabled soldiers in Veterans Administration hospitals. Today over 5,000 music therapists work in clinical settings throughout the United States.

Music as therapy, however, has deeper roots. Early Egyptian tomb paintings display musicians accompanying the deceased to enhance the afterlife (Figure 31). Ancient Greek thinkers, such as Aristotle and Pythagoras, believed that music could facilitate healing. "Singing" is a part of Native American healing rituals that are hundreds of years old (see Chapter 5). Incantations and chants are part of many shamanic traditions, and are included in the oldest references to medical practices.

Music therapy is used as a complementary therapy for many diseases in a wide variety of clinical settings, including hospitals, rehabilitation centers, and nursing homes. Music therapists work with all patient groups, including premature infants, the terminally ill, and patients with substance abuse problems, mental illness, chronic pain, physical disabilities, brain injuries, Alzheimer's disease and other forms of dementia, and childhood developmental disabilities such as mental retardation and autism.

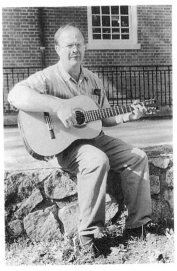

Figure 30 Music therapy is practiced in many forms, including actively playing instruments and listening to recordings.

What Practitioners Say It Does

Music therapy has several purposes. It can alleviate pain and ease the psychological discomfort associated with many medical conditions. It helps improve physical and mental functioning of people with neurological or developmental disorders.

Therapists say that music therapy can help terminally ill patients decrease anxiety, depression, and pain, and improve their quality of life. It helps reduce the need for medication among patients and during childbirth, and distracts dental patients from the pain of root canal. It can improve the ability of mentally handicapped and autistic children to learn, to interact with other people, and to relate to their environments. It enhances the well-being of elderly patients in nursing homes, including those suffering dementia.

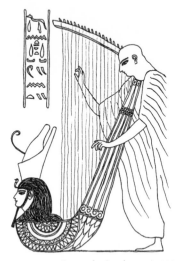

Figure 31 The enduring importance of music is illustrated in this copy of an Egyptian tomb painting.

Beliefs on Which It Is Based

There is no single theory to explain how music therapy works in various clinical situations. Instead, music therapists offer explanatory hypotheses for different settings. In addition, despite substantial research on music therapy, the mechanisms by which it works in healing are not well understood.

In reducing pain, music therapy may act as the relaxation response does in meditation (see Chapter 18). Soothing music has been shown to reduce blood pressure, breathing rates, and other aspects of physiological functions. Altering physiological activity may both provide distraction from pain and promote relaxation.

Music therapy for stroke victims and patients with other neurological deficits may work through **entrainment**. As patients listen to music that has a consistent beat, their muscle movements come to synchronize with the beat. Motions become increasingly efficient and regular, which in turn improves the ability to walk and develop other motor skills. In essence, it is believed that practicing motor skills to a rhythm hones those skills and makes them more efficient.

Research Evidence to Date

Music therapy has been subjected to a great deal of research during the past three decades, and several professional journals are devoted to music therapy. Although many published articles consist of descriptions and anecdotal evidence, larger, more organized studies have also been conducted. These studies indicate that music therapy can be an effective complementary technique for various medical conditions.

Premature babies exposed to music in intensive-care units gain weight more quickly and are discharged more quickly than babies who do not hear music. Music therapy also has been shown to reduce anxiety levels in children undergoing surgical and medical procedures. Research supports the ability of music therapy to increase retarded children's motor skills and assist their capacity to learn math and other subjects. It has been used successfully to strengthen coordination and walking skills among children with muscular or skeletal disorders, to improve the speech of hearing-impaired

The Alternative Medicine Handbook

students, and to lessen the isolation of autism.

Studies of music therapy with Alzheimer's patients and other victims of dementia reveal that musical cues increase patients' attention and ability to focus on their surroundings. Music therapy also reduces the agitation that often accompanies Alzheimer's disease. Working with Alzheimer's patients in nursing homes, music therapists help patients perform simple group exercises such as beating a drum in time with the rest of the group, or they may work one-on-one with patients, playing songs that have been significant in the patients' lives. In both group and individual activities, patients who are not normally responsive to speech or who do not recognize friends and relatives can become responsive for a time and connect with their immediate surroundings.

Music reduces the amount of anesthesia required during labor. It is the practice in some hospitals to have pregnant women select music to accompany their labor. Women often choose different music for each stage. During labor, they can use a remote control to regulate volume.

Music therapy also reduces self-reported levels of dental and postoperative pain. It assists the physical rehabilitation of patients with stroke and Parkinson's disease, improving the rate at which patients learn to walk when compared with no-music-therapy control patients. Stroke victims receiving music therapy also have reported lower levels of anxiety and higher scores on measures of psychological health when compared with control groups. Several small studies have shown that music therapy can improve speech among those with traumatic brain injuries. Researchers at the University of California at Irvine produced evidence that listening to Mozart produced short-term enhancement of spatial-temporal reasoning abilities in college students.

Current government-supported initiatives in music therapy include a focus on patients with brain injuries and on the aged. In 1992, Congress passed an act that provided $1 million in annual funding for music therapy research and education with elderly patients.

What It Can Do for You

Music therapy is a documented, effective complementary therapy for many conditions and problems. It is not a curative treatment, nor is it promoted, as are some other complementary therapies, as a cure for serious diseases. As do the best of complementary treatments, however, it can improve well-being and quality of life, reduce symptoms, and enhance the effectiveness of primary treatment and rehabilitation therapy.

Music therapy is especially desirable because, for most people, it is an intrinsically pleasant, soothing experience. Furthermore, it is noninvasive, free of danger or side effects, usable in almost any setting and with any other treatment, and inexpensive. Music therapy appears to be an underutilized, extremely helpful complementary technique.

If you think you or a member of your family have a problem that may benefit from music therapy, ask your primary caregiver if they know of music therapists who work with that condition, or contact an organization listed in the following section.

Where to Get It

There are two professional organizations for music therapists: the National Association for Music Therapy (NAMT), with more than 3,200 members, and the American Association for Music Therapy (AAMT), which has over 500 members. These two organizations plan to merge in the near future.

+ The National Association is located in Silver Spring, Maryland (301 589-3300), and can be found on the World Wide Web (http://www.namt.com/namt).
+ The American Association is located in Ossining, New York (914 944-9260).
+ Both organizations can provide general information about music therapy, about universities with music therapy programs in your area, and about qualified music therapists near your home. (The Certification Board for Music Therapists was established in 1983.) Often, music therapists specialize in specific patient groups, working, for example, with palliative care teams to help terminally ill patients, or treating developmentally challenged children.

There appear to be two distinct categories of sound therapy. One category includes the broadly recognized, commonsensical notion that pleasant sounds make us feel calm, while jarring sounds startle us into unpleasant moods. "Therapeutic" sound, therefore, would be peaceful, unobtrusive, pleasant.

The second category includes broader and more serious promises for sound, including claims that it can influence and heal internal organs. Alternative sound therapy is a New Age combination of mysticism and sacred healing incantations. It entails many claims, none of which are proven or even discussed in the medical or scientific literature.

From a scientist's perspective, sound is created by the vibration of objects, which causes the air to move in waves. Individual sounds have different frequencies, and frequencies determine the sound's pitch (the greater the frequency, the higher the pitch). Intensity or volume are other qualities of sound. The often pleasing sound of a bird chirping creates sound waves that are close together, which increases their frequency and produces high-pitched sounds, while the sound of a frightening thunderclap, with great intensity, creates waves of a much lower frequency and therefore deeper sound. Sound enters the body not only through the auditory system, beginning with the ear, but also as vibrations on other parts of the body such as the skull.

Sound tapes are created to produce special responses in listeners. The sounds of a spring rainstorm or ocean waves lapping against a beach are marketed in the form of audiocassettes and CDs to provide a pleasing, relaxing background that can reduce stress and promote relaxation. **White sound** machines obliterate other sounds and neutralize the auditory environment. Many people use them to aid sleep.

Proponents of sound therapy believe that various types of sound can have specific therapeutic effects on the mind and body. Based on the known physiological impact of sound waves, or vibrations, sound therapists have devised methods for focusing these vibrations on

Enhancing Well-Being through the Senses

particular areas of the body and on specific organs for therapeutic purposes.

What It Is

Sound therapy uses sound from a variety of human-made sources to improve emotional or physical status. Several different approaches promote these beneficial effects. **Toning**, for example, is a technique in which the subject produces elongated vowel sounds in an effort to eliminate stress. This technique also is said to improve the speaking and singing voice. It is thought helpful because vowel-sound vibrations are assumed to resonate therapeutically through the entire body.

A trademarked process called "Biosonic Repatterning" uses **cymatics**—defined as the science of wave phenomena—in combination with toning and healing **mantras** (sacred incantations) to activate "elemental energy qualities." This combination is said to reestablish healthy resonance in tissues. Tuning forks, because of their perfect pitch and vibrations, may also be involved in this New Age amalgam of sound-wave phenomena and ancient, unprovable concepts of vital internal energy.

Pain management through the use of a sound-producing instrument called the **Infratonic QGM**, invented by a Chinese scientist to replicate secondary sound waves created by masters of *qigong*, is another and related application of sound therapy. Similarly, a process called **Sonopuncture** involves combining ultrasound with acupoints. (**Ultrasound** is more commonly known as a modern diagnostic device that uses sound waves to study internal body structures and organs.) Sonopuncture sometimes is applied along with vibration devices, toning, Biosonic Repatterning, and other alternative therapies.

Alfred A. Tomatis, M.D., a Paris physician and teacher, developed an instrument called the **electronic ear**, which is said to modify sound frequencies and train the ear to hear a broader range of frequencies. Sound therapists use this device to teach patients how to focus on sounds and listen more effectively.

Another French physician, Guy Berard, believed that behavioral and cognitive problems can be caused by distortions in certain perceived sound frequencies. He developed a device known as **EERS**, an acronym for Ears Education and Retraining System, that would filter and modify aberrant frequencies to correct sound-related disorders.

What Practitioners Say It Does

Soothing sounds are claimed to promote deep relaxation and meditation. Sometimes unusual techniques are applied. For example, ethereal sounds are said to be produced by thirty-five crystal bowls played on an "armonica," a contemporary instrument claimed to be created from an extinct invention of Benjamin Franklin.

Instruments that transmit sounds through the skin (**cymatic therapy**) are promoted to stimulate natural regulatory and immunologic systems. Practitioners claim that sound therapy in the form of "rapid acoustic stimuli" helps children with dyslexia. It is also claimed to help those with attention deficit disorder and other learning dysfunctions. The effectiveness of sound therapy is said to increase when used in conjunction with acupuncture.

All of these claims are supported only by anecdotal reports; they remain unproven.

Beliefs on Which It Is Based

Proponents of sound therapy believe that rhythms of the heart, brain, and other organs are synchronous, and that illness occurs when these rhythms are disturbed. They also believe that external rhythmic stimuli can override the natural rhythm of heartbeats and cause the heart to beat in time with that external rhythm.

The proven kernel of scientific accuracy is that soothing music, an external rhythmic stimulus, can reduce heart rate and relax the body, just as loud, jarring sounds can induce a startle reaction and increase heart rate. Sound therapy concepts, other than those related to music, have not been tested scientifically and are not discussed in the medical literature.

Research Evidence to Date

Although some small studies have been conducted, they lack the necessary scientific rigor to supply any verification. Virtually none of these studies have appeared in medical or scientific journals in the last thirty years. Cymatic therapy, for all its quasi-medical claims, is not listed in standard medical dictionaries, journals, or textbooks.

What It Can Do for You

The use of pleasing sounds as a background for work or relaxation, and in stressful environments such as dentists' offices, can produce the kind of positive results that most of us have experienced. Waves lapping on a beach, wind gently rustling leaves, soft rain, forest bird calls—these are examples of soothing sounds. When pleasing sounds help us relax, our heart rate slows and we feel better. Exposure to noise or harsh sound, on the other hand, causes unwanted stress.

Claims that sound therapy can cure disease are unfounded.

Where to Get It

+ *Roar of Silence*, by Don Campbell (Theosophical Publishing House, Wheaton, Ill., 1989).
+ *The Conscious Ear*, by Alfred Tomatis (Staton Hill Books, Tarrytown, N.Y., 1991).
+ *Sound Health*, by Steven Halpern (Harper Collins Publishers, New York, 1985).
+ *Rhythms of Learning*, by Don Campbell (Zephyr Press Learning Materials, Tucson, 1991).

The Sound Listening and Learning Center in Phoenix, Arizona (602 381-0086), and the Sound Healers Association and Spirit Music in Boulder, Colorado (303 443-8181), can supply information.

RESTORING HEALTH WITH EXTERNAL ENERGY FORCES

Belief in the existence of an external energy force that we can not only capture but control for our own purposes is as old as the history of medicine itself. Spirits, magic, deities, and other all-powerful forces were once thought to control the universe and its components.

In fact, the space around us is filled with all manner of electromagnetic energy, forms of external energy that the ancients could not have imagined. Modern science also has shown that cells of the human body, like all matter, emit electrical charges, although they are extremely small charges.

Many previously inexplicable natural events, such as birth, the waning moon, or the eruption of volcanos, are now understood and much more predictable. When answers to questions about illness elude us, however, it is not surprising that we turn again to the old spiritual, physical, or even magical external forces to search for cause and cure, and sometimes to the more recently understood wonders of electromagnetic energy fields. Although the several alternative and complementary approaches discussed in this part differ profoundly from one another in significant ways, their practitioners share the belief that external energy forces, whether from the human body, electromagnetic fields, or the energy of faith and spirituality, contain important healing capacities.

Crystal healing is a New Age version of the ancient belief that stones harbor magical healing energy. Stones of different hues are thought to produce particular results or attack specific ailments. Lovely and simple to use (you just hold them or place them on your body or around the room), they are the most whimsical of the "external healing forces" included in this section. Perhaps because they refract light in what originally must have been inexplicable ways, crystals were assumed to hold special energy. Ironically, quartz, a common crystal long imbued with imaginary curative powers, is now a source of power in the form of silicon dioxide chips, the energy-transmitting heart of computer technology.

The history of electromagnetic therapies parallels the discovery of electricity and its use in modern society. When it was understood that different frequencies operating at varying levels of power produced different effects, opportunists and entrepreneurs in substantial numbers found ways to apply those variations to the "diagnosis" and "treatment" of illness and other problems. As products failed to produce benefits (such as the electric hairbrush sold to eliminate baldness), they were dropped, quickly to be replaced by yet other products that relied on the newly discovered miracle of electric power.

Today, electric energy is used in important diagnostic and treatment technologies, such as X rays to diagnose illness, to restart stopped hearts, and to help repair broken bones. Some alternative practitioners use weak electromagnetic fields as therapy for cancer and other major ailments, but these applications remain unproven.

In a very different application of external energy for healing purposes, some advocates use their own energy to heal others. They claim to send their internal healing energy into the body of another by passing their hands several inches over that person in what is called "therapeutic touch." Healers also use heat, moxibustion, acupuncture, and other external means to influence the patient's own internal energy and health, applying "energy therapy" in the process.

Probably the most frequently called upon system of healing energy is prayer and spirituality. Although prayer and spirituality could be discussed in many contexts in addition to that of external energy forces, they do involve reaching out beyond the self to a greater force for help in times of illness and despair. Prayers have been used by mankind for thousands of years, directed at various magical powers and deities. Modern prayers around the world today are often directed toward a single, all powerful deity, typically asking for assistance to bring about a healthier or better life for the supplicant. Beyond belief in all-powerful external beings, the basis of prayer rests on the belief that a deity is able and potentially willing to intervene, to respond to requests for assistance, and to cure disease.

Once prayer became an established practice, faith healers came forth to proclaim their unique ability to communicate with God and to use their special powers to cure disease and illness. Faith healers have existed in cultures around the world and throughout history. Some take advantage of their constituents, using fakery and deceit. Nevertheless, people continue to seek them out, particularly when mainstream medicine cannot cure their problems but sometimes in place of medical care that is readily obtainable. Some faith healers use television pulpits. Others preach their gospel in tent revival meetings, traveling from city to city.

Shamans, religious leaders, or priests of earlier times were revered by their communities for their mystical abilities to cure the sick. Shamanism began as early as 20,000 to 40,000 years ago, when medicine, magic, and religion were inextricably combined. Shamans were believed able to communicate with ancestral spirits and gods, beings who remained unseen and unheard by ordinary people. Shamans used their external power to heal the ailments of individuals, reverse the inequities of nature, and manage the problems of the community.

Contemporary shamans work in today's Native American and other indigenous cultures. Often, however, their repertoire of curative powers now includes some modern and conventional medical practices, and they may collaborate with mainstream physicians.

Perhaps one day science will provide the answers to pressing questions about disease prevention, diagnosis, and cure that continue to plague humankind. That level of insight would profoundly change some of the approaches discussed in this section. However, it is likely that some approaches—such as spirituality, the enjoyment of nature's crystalline beauty, and increasingly advanced applications of electromagnetism—will remain integral components of human civilization.

A basic rule of nature is that energy is produced by the breakdown of matter. Fire is a good example. It produces heat and light as its fuel is consumed. Minerals, including crystals and gems, produce no energy except for those few that are radioactive. Radioactive minerals break down and convert their own substance into inert minerals. Quartz crystal is not radioactive. Inert and chemically stable, it neither produces energy nor vibrates. It just sits there, looking beautiful, mysterious, and inscrutable.

Silicon chips used in computers transmit energy only because energy is put through them. They serve as a vehicle for externally infused energy. Quartz is silicon dioxide, and ground-up quartz is sand. Both quartz and sand are abundant and common on this earth. Quartz is a hexagonal (six-sided) crystal. Despite its abundance, quartz is the most popular of New Age stones, and despite its total absence of energy or magnetism, New Agers believe it has these and other characteristics. Crystal healing is based on the incorrect idea that crystals contain energy that can restore health, promote growth, provide protection, and guide people to the "spiritual" world of the soul.

What It Is

Crystal healing involves very simple procedures, such as placing particular stones around one's home, carrying them in a pocket, wearing them around the neck or elsewhere as ornaments, and touching them as the urge arises. In more formal types of crystal healing, a healer places various colored stones on different parts of the body. Often these are the body spots identified as meridians in traditional Chinese medicine (see Chapter 3) and known as chakras in ancient India's Ayurvedic medicine (see Chapter 2).

New Agers also believe that different colors have particular therapeutic value. Red-orange agate, for example, is thought to energize, amethyst is said to calm the conscious and subconscious mind (Figure 32), and bloodstone (or heliotrope) is believed to purify the blood.

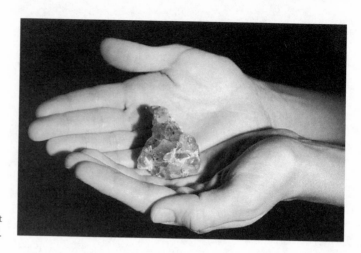

Figure 32 The violet amethyst
is said to calm the mind.

Furthermore, the type of crystals used plays a role in the healing performed. Malachite is thought to help uncover emotional traumas associated with the heart chakra, while smoky quartz helps generate vibrations at the top of the head (the "crown chakra" in Ayurvedic medicine). The patterns, colors, and type of a given crystal, along with incantations and other rituals, also influence healing.

What Practitioners Say It Does

Most crystal healers do not make direct health claims, such as "malachite cures heart disease." Rather, they claim that crystals cure the underlying defects in thoughts and emotions of which physical disease is a symptom. Physical illness is perceived as an important sign that one's mental, emotional, or physical status is not in alignment with "the light," the divine energy that underlies all creation and places the user in touch with universal consciousness. By bringing the body back into alignment with the light, illness is said to be cured.

Many claims made for crystals are not related to physical health at all, but instead concern such features as auras, etheric wisdom, and past lives. The mythology of crystals includes their ability to foretell the future and reveal the past. Some subscribe to the idea that crystals connect us with almost forgotten sources of ancient wisdom, kindly left for our eventual enlightenment by alien beings now departed from our world.

The Alternative Medicine Handbook

Beliefs on Which It Is Based

The idea behind crystal healing is simply that crystals have powers. The notion is ancient and enduring. However, the magical powers attributed to crystals by the ancients are known to be physical phenomena that can be explained by the basic laws of physics or that have been discarded by science as properties that simply do not exist.

Many ancient cultures, including the Greeks, Egyptians, Babylonians, and Asians, believed crystals to have powers or to serve as homes for spirits. Crystals were believed to house angels, demons, or fairies. At one point in the Old Testament, God is said to dwell in a stone. In Sanskrit terminology, spirits inside crystals were known as *devas*, or gods.

In ancient times, people believed that crystals gave off light. The ancient Hindus thought that the underworld was illuminated by huge gems, acting as minor suns. The Greeks had similar beliefs. According to medieval legend, the very top of the Church of the Holy Grail held a huge light-emitting ruby, serving as a beacon to guide the Grail knights.

Research Evidence to Date

Belief in the light-emitting powers of crystals is understandable but wrong. Fluorescent or phosphorescent minerals appear to give off light. However, the source of the light is outside the crystals themselves. Fluorescent crystals reflect ultraviolet light that is invisible to the naked eye, while phosphorescent crystals retain and reemit light for a period of time after the original light source has ended.

No formal research on the healing powers of crystals has been conducted. The absence of scientific studies is appropriate given the fanciful nature and lack of rationale for these beliefs. The idea that crystals and other stones hold special powers is a part of ancient mythology, resurrected in the West in recent years.

Even ardent alternative-healing proponents do not take crystal "healing" seriously. Indeed, the very comprehensive and detailed report of the Office of Alternative Medicine makes no mention of crystal healing.

What It Can Do For You

The mythical superstitions associated with crystal healing—the auras, nonphysical planes of existence, magical energy, past lives, and so on—are not real and therefore have no effect on health and illness. Crystals do not heal. With that understanding, and so long as one maintains a recreational spirit, collecting stones has rewards and benefits. For some, playing with crystals is simply the focus of an occasional foray into the enchanting world of mystery and make-believe. Others find that stroking stones or lying comfortably with them, especially when accompanied by meditation, feels relaxing and helps reduce stress.

Many are delighted by the beauty and agelessness of crystals. And of course, collecting stones can be a rewarding, enlightening, and interesting hobby. Perhaps those who benefit most from people's interest in crystal healing are the shopkeepers who sell "magic" crystals, which are sold at much higher prices than nonmagic crystals. However, the two types are identical in every respect.

Where to Get It

Occult shops, New Age haunts, and some health-food stores sell magic stones. But the same stones are available at far less expense from hobby and mineral shops.

⮑50
Electro-magnetic Therapies

The biological effects of magnetism, and of what eventually was identified as electricity, have been studied since the time of early Greek and Roman civilizations. It is believed that **lodestones**, pieces of naturally occurring minerals with magnetic properties, were found eons ago when people literally stumbled upon them.

By the eleventh and twelfth centuries, lodestones were thought to have curative powers and were used to treat gout, arthritis, baldness, and other ailments, as described by medieval writers. Scholars of the time also believed that magnets could cause and cure melancholy. Aphrodisiac powers were attributed to lodestones probably because of their "magnetic" ability to attract.

Along with the magical ideas, magnets were applied to solve practical problems such as locating shattered knife blades and other iron objects in wounded people. A century later, the Swiss physician Paracelsus studied magnets as a possible treatment for epilepsy.

Franz Mesmer, an eighteenth-century Viennese physician, developed a theory of "animal magnetism," which he believed to be a basic biophysical force similar to gravity and capable of profound neuropsychiatric and physical effects. His first scientific treatise on this topic, *On the Medicinal Uses of the Magnet*, was published in 1775. Although he credited his successful treatment of a woman with numerous complaints to a magnet's ability to realign polarity in her internal organs, it soon became clear that he had discovered hypnotism instead (hence the word *mesmerize*). "Animal magnetism" was shown later to be not the claimed biophysical force, but a reaction to the power of suggestion. (For the use of hypnosis in healing, see Chapter 15.)

Interest in the therapeutic potential of both electricity and magnets persisted throughout history, with most ideas and products eventually deemed pure quackery. The nineteenth century, called by medical historians the "golden age of medical electricity," was also known as the "electromagnetic era of medical quackery." A popular and typical electromagnetic device called the I-ON-A-CO was sold in the late 1920s by Gaylord Wilshire (for

Restoring Health with External Energy Forces

whom Hollywood's Wilshire Boulevard was named). It was shaped like a large horse collar and worn over the shoulders to cure any ailment that might arise. It didn't work.

As science learned more about electricity, entrepreneurs developed parallel alternative systems: a variety of "black boxes" connected to electrical sources were promoted as "energy-healing" devices, or as "vibrational medicine." Less than a century ago, advertisements touting electronic cure-alls were prevalent in U.S. newspapers and magazines. A broad variety of electric and magnetic instruments were marketed, sometimes at outrageous prices, to compete with mainstream medicine for the treatment of many ailments. Electronic devices, including the Auto Electronic Radioclast, Electron-O-Ray, Depoloray, and many others, were promoted as cures for cancer and other diseases. They were marketed into the 1990s.

The manufacture and distribution of such quasi-medical devices eventually were regulated by the Food, Drug and Cosmetic Act (FDCA), enforced by the Food and Drug Administration (FDA). In 1976, a Medical Devices Amendment to the Food, Drug and Cosmetic Act was enacted. It required proper labeling of medical devices and the restriction of claims to those that could be proven. Some devices, such as powerful magnets sold to cure cancer, continue to be marketed, skirting the regulations by careful wording of curative claims.

What It Is

As in all matter, electricity exists within our bodies at extremely low levels. Brain waves are produced on an electro-encephalogram (EEG), and the rhythm of heartbeats can be recorded on an electrocardiogram (EKG or ECG). These diagnostic tools depend on electricity emitted by the brain and heart, respectively, to produce "pictures" of activity in those organs.

Electricity in varying frequencies and strengths is used in mainstream medicine for certain therapeutic purposes. Perhaps the most dramatic application occurs in the hospital emergency room, where two highly charged paddles, applied against a patient's chest, transmit a jolt of electricity to the body in order to restart a stopped heart.

Electromagnetic therapy

It is called by many names: bioelectricity, electronic devices, electromagnetism, biomagnetism, magnetobiology (in the former USSR), electromagnetic or magnetic field therapy, and magnetic healing.

The theoretic thread that seems to bind these approaches is the fact that the body does emit a slight magnetic field of its own.

Low-frequency electric current is used to speed the healing of some bone fractures. The current speeds growth of osteoblasts, the cells that develop into bone, and these cells knit the broken parts together. Radiation therapy uses yet another type of electrical force to treat cancer. **TENS (transcutaneous electrical nerve stimulation)** units help treat certain types of pain and neurological disorders. Some acupuncturists send low-level electrical stimulation through acupuncture needles to enhance their effect.

Although most electromagnetic devices of the past have been deemed useless, consumer interest continues to support their availability. Often, an apparatus serves as a source of electrical or magnetic energy, typically using extremely low intensity fields.

Alternative electromagnetic therapies usually employ galvanic devices such as the Ellis Micro-Dynameter to diagnose and treat disease. These instruments use two electrodes of different metals to measure electric current. The electrodes often are applied to two acupuncture points to identify areas of inflammation, irritation, or degeneration. Practitioners of electromagnetic therapies believe that electrical resistance on the skin indicates the health of body organs. Measured by galvanic devices, variations from a "norm" are used to diagnose disease. In actuality, electrodes placed on the skin simply measure changes in the electrical resistance of the skin, not events inside the body.

Scientific knowledge of the human body, electricity, and magnetism, sometimes combined with unsubstantiated concepts of an energy "life force," form the basis for the deductive leap made by some practitioners to the claim that electromagnetic therapy can heal virtually any illness.

Alternative electromagnetic therapies remain unproven and cannot be accepted with the same assurance afforded mainstream medicine's well-documented use of electrotherapies.

What Practitioners Say It Does

Contemporary claims for alternative uses of electricity as therapy have not been substantiated. Most advocates today promote the ability of electromagnetism to

Magnetism in Humans

Each molecule in the human body contains a tiny amount of magnetic energy. Magnetism is closely related to electricity, and electric currents generate magnetic fields.

Men's brain cells are said to have stronger magnetic fields than women's. Scientists believe this may explain why most men are better able than most women to find their way around and to differentiate directions of the compass.

stimulate tissue regeneration or enhance the immune system through the use of external electrical energy sources. Electrical overstimulation of muscles is said to promote relaxation, thus improving oxygen and nutrient supply, waste removal, and the strengthening of treated muscles. These are unproven claims.

Electric current and electromagnetic field applications are used by some practitioners to treat ulcers, burns, nerve and spinal cord injuries, diabetes, gum infections in dentistry, asthma, heart disease, and other maladies. One type of therapy involves placing an antenna in the patient's mouth, through which low-level electromagnetic energy is administered to treat insomnia and hypertension. A magnetic pulse generator is used in lieu of electroconvulsive therapy (informally known as electroshock) to treat depression and seizures.

In Russia, where modern medications and therapies are available to very few, extensive use of **microwave resonance therapy** with low-intensity microwave radiation continues as an unproven treatment for arthritis, ulcers, chronic pain, nerve disorders, cerebral palsy, and other diseases. In the Western world, magnetic devices, sometimes fashioned as bracelets, belts, or tiny discs contained in adhesive bandages, are promoted to achieve pain relief. Larger "super magnets" are still promoted as cancer cures.

Scientific data do not support the effectiveness of magnetic or electric fields in these alternative methods of diagnosis or treatment of disease. It is ironic that electromagnetic therapies are being promoted today as alternative cures for cancer and other diseases, since international scientific research is simultaneously examining the possibility that even very weak electromagnetic fields can promote cancer in some body cells.

Beliefs on Which It Is Based

Scientifically, it is known that the human body is regulated by electrical forces, and that it cannot function without its own internal electrical energy system. The heart beats as a result of contractions triggered by electrical impulses, and the nervous system regulates body systems, movement, and thought through a combination of chemical and electrical stimuli. Each molecule in our body has its own minute magnetic and electrical force. We cannot survive without the extremely low levels of electricity that regulate and sustain life within us.

Those who practice alternative electromagnetic therapies, however, go beyond accepted scientific knowledge, believing that disease and illness are caused when electrical energy within our bodies becomes imbalanced or misaligned. Some practitioners further believe that the electric devices they have developed can supply electrical energy to the body or to a specific organ within the body and correct the "imbalances" that are claimed to cause disease.

There is another belief that bioelectric energy may simply carry or transmit "information" necessary to cell life. This hypothesized mechanism is used to explain the workings of homeopathic medicine (see Chapter 4), in which medications are so diluted that no molecule of the original product remains. Proponents believe that the "information" originally contained in the dissolved material remains as a trace memory in the form of bioelectric energy in the solution. This bioelectric energy "memory" is thought to provide the promised therapeutic benefit.

Research Evidence to Date

The need for the body's own electricity to sustain life is documented through scientific investigation and discovery. Its roles in regulating the heartbeat and maintaining the neuromuscular system are well documented. Low-level electric current is known to stimulate the healing of bone fractures. Radiation therapy, magnetic resonance imaging (MRI), and X rays are among the established scientific applications of electricity in mainstream medicine.

The marketing of unproven "black box" approaches to electromagnetic therapy has been restrained by the FDA. These devices, variations of which have been sold for decades, have been examined and are considered completely bogus.

What It Can Do for You

Mainstream medicine's use of electricity in its many applications is extremely helpful. Indeed, in the emergency room, it saves lives. But the application of electric currents and magnetic fields to cure disease as promised by alternative practitioners remains unproven.

Beyond mainstream medicine, there is little convincing evidence that externally applied electrical forces can improve health or cure disease.

Where to Get It

Electrical stimulation is used extensively by many acupuncturists, physical therapists, and rehabilitation therapists. Some cosmetologists now use electrically stimulated acupuncture to strengthen facial muscles. However, there is scant evidence that the many alternative applications of bioelectromagnetic energy that rise and fall in popularity over time are effective or useful. Despite the absence of documented benefit, these devices are used or sold by many chiropractors, naturopaths, acupuncturists, and marketers of various unproven and disproved remedies, including electric devices. Should you be drawn to try electromagnetic therapy, consult your physician first.

Information about electric and magnetic fields (EMF) research is provided in a booklet produced by the U.S. Department of Energy. Called *EMF in the Workplace*, the booklet is available at no cost and may be obtained by calling the federal government EMF Infoline at (800) 363-2383.

The National Institute of Environmental Health Sciences also has information about the effects of electromagnetic currents:

✦ NIEHS
P.O. Box 1233
Research Triangle Park, NC 27709
Telephone: (919) 541-3345

$\sim$51
Faith Healing

In the first book of Corinthians in the New Testament, the gifts bestowed on the faithful by the Holy Spirit are enumerated. One of these is the "gift of healing" (I Corinthians 12:9). Although this refers most significantly to the spiritual ability to draw the good out of suffering, it also refers to the ability to bring about physical healing. In the almost two millennia since the time this was written, various people and places have gained reputations for their power to heal. They claim to have the miraculous capacity to banish illness through faith.

In medieval times, the doctrine of the divine right of kings espoused that monarchs could heal by the laying on of their royal hands. St. Catherine of Siena and other saints throughout history also were believed to have the power to heal. In modern times, some evangelists as well as others have claimed similar gifts. The Christian Science Church, for example, believes that its practitioners and nurses can cure illness through prayer.

Today, the term *faith healer* is most frequently used to identify those people who claim to have a special power derived from God that enables them to cure illness and disease. Faith-healing ceremonies typically are conducted in an atmosphere of high emotion, often on television or in traveling revival meetings, by self-appointed, religiously inspired "healers."

The term *faith healing* is applied also to a variety of efforts aimed at eliminating disease and disability through prayer, through visiting a religious shrine, or simply through an individual's strong belief in a Supreme Being. Sometimes these activities occur in the presence of a priest from an organized religion who leads the patient and family in more traditional prayer.

Strong opinions exist on both sides of the debate about the power of faith healers and the ability of prayer to cure sickness and disease. Contemporary thinkers continue to debate the possibility that a combination of the patient's faith in a higher power and the healer's ability to capture and transmit that power to the patient can cure disease.

What It Is

There appear to be three distinct phenomena involved

in faith healing: the claims of faith healers that miraculous cures are possible, the influence that mind and belief can have on health and disease (the placebo effect), and the fact of spontaneous remissions, which occur rarely but regularly in medicine. When evaluating the claims of faith healers, it is important to consider and distinguish among these three factors.

Faith healing is the idea that someone or something can eliminate disease or dysfunction in another individual. It is offered by people who claim to have a special gift themselves or who claim that particular locations, such as the famous French shrine at Lourdes, are imbued with the power to heal. Faith healing is said to occur also through the power of prayer on the part of the patient or through others praying for the patient's recovery.

The **placebo effect** (see Chapter 19) describes the therapeutic effect of inert substances that derives from the patient's belief that the substance is beneficial. In drug studies it is well known that 30 to 40 percent, and possibly up to 80 or 90 percent of patients show improvement solely as a result of placebo interventions. Finally, there have been documented cases of "miraculous" cures, unexpected recoveries, and spontaneous remissions from diseases such as cancer and conditions such as coma that cannot be explained by medical science.

What Practitioners Say It Does

Faith healers claim they can cure virtually all problems. This includes physical disabilities such as blindness and deafness, serious illness such as cancer and AIDS, and developmental disorders.

The scope of faith healing reflects the medical knowledge of the time. In the Middle Ages, for example, kings were believed to be capable of curing tuberculosis, then called scrofula. Today, tuberculosis can be prevented and treated by conventional medicine, and faith healers no longer attempt to cure it. As with other forms of alternative medicine, faith healing tends to offer hope for conditions that conventional medicine cannot cure or treat effectively at that point in time.

Beliefs on Which It Is Based

Faith healing rests on three core beliefs:

1. A power, which may be a god or a psychic force, can be accessed by the healing agent;
2. The healing agent can not only access this power, but also use it to heal disease;
3. The faith of the patient is essential. Failures in faith healing often are attributed not to the shortcomings of the healer, but to a lack of faith on the part of the patient.

Most scientists view faith healing as a means of eliciting the placebo effect. Believing that it can cure often imbues a medication, person, institution, incantation, or prayer with curative power. For the vast majority of serious problems, however, faith healing disappoints. It fails to produce the expected results for which many patients pay great sums of money. (Of course, the same may be said about many medical therapies).

Research Evidence to Date

Probably the most serious and thorough modern investigations of faith healing have been conducted by James Randi, author of the book *The Faith Healers*. Randi has debunked television evangelists by exposing hidden microphones and other means of communication through which backstage conspirators provide information to the on-air healer. Similarly, he has shown that "paralyzed" people who magically rise from their wheelchairs after apparent successful faith healing actually are ambulatory individuals acting the part.

Randi reports that the modern faith healers he studied are either sincere but misguided and unable to produce healing, or outright charlatans and quacks who rely on trickery to impress the frightened and gullible.

Randi not only uncovers the tricks used by faith healers, but also describes the logical fallacies that many use to make it difficult to disprove faith healing. Most illnesses, for example, run a natural course, at the end of which the patient's health returns. If faith healing is attempted during this time, the patient's eventual and inevitable improvement is attributed by the healer to the "faith healing." Alternately, lack of improvement following a faith-healing effort typically is attributed to lack of faith, or inadequate faith, on the part of the patient. This removes the onus of proof from the healer.

Spontaneous remission from cancer has been the subject of many studies. Despite research efforts, spontaneous remissions remain a poorly understood phenomenon of natural biology. No consistent set of physiological, psychological, religious, or demographic characteristics are associated with people who experience spontaneous remissions. Original work in this field revealed that approximately one in 100,000 cancer patients experiences unexpected remission. Of the approximately 1.2 million new cases of cancer diagnosed in the United States each year, twelve spontaneous remissions would be expected statistically.

There is a commission of the Roman Catholic Church that authenticates the miracles said to occur at the famous Lourdes shrine. Numerous miraculous cures are claimed by the approximately one hundred million visitors to the shrine. The Church committee, however, using its extremely strict guidelines, has rejected the authenticity of most, and validated only 65 miracle cures in the 150 years since people have flocked to this shrine. Given the number of visitors over that period of time, this number of "miraculous cures" is far fewer than the expected rate of spontaneous remission.

What It Can Do For You

Unfortunately, the history of faith healing and healers seems to contain many more stories of charlatans fleecing the unwary than of true miracles. However, although it has never restored missing limbs and although it rarely dissipates serious physiological disease, faith and religious belief, possibly through the placebo effect, can produce important health benefits. These include the relief of pain and anxiety, and possibly the prolonging of life so that an individual lives until a personally important anniversary.

The study of seeming "miracle" cures such as spontaneous remissions may one day produce information that will help fight disease.

Where to Get It

The history of faith healers reveals that many have been exposed as unscrupulous. There is no evidence that healing can be purchased. Religious belief and faith in and of themselves may be valuable and worthwhile for many, but the extravagant claims of some healers can trap the unwary.

The Alternative Medicine Handbook

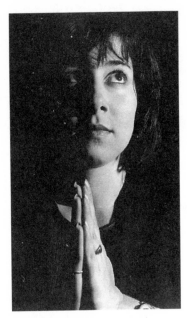

52
Prayer and Spirituality

Religion has been an integral component of the human community since the beginning of recorded history. From the 30,000-year-old Venus figure icons of fertility prayer (see the introduction to Part I), to the gods of ancient Egypt and Greece, to modern Christianity, Judaism, Islam, Hinduism, and Buddhism—every culture at each period of time and in every corner of this globe developed systems of religion and spirituality. Some manner of prayer served as the institutionalized means of seeking assistance from a being or beings believed sufficiently powerful to alter nature, the elements, health, and disease.

Prayers have been uttered for the prosperity, safety, physical and spiritual well-being, good weather, and bountiful harvests for the living and to help the souls of the dead. The scope of prayer is limited only by the scope of human desire and enterprise. The power of prayer to influence illness and health has become the subject of intense scientific inquiry. Can prayer have a medical effect? Are those who hold religious beliefs physically healthier than those who do not? Some recent studies claim that prayer can have a positive effect on health, although critics point to serious shortcomings in the research methods employed. Some groups now advocate prayer as a complement to medical therapy, while others, such as the Christian Science Church, use it in place of conventional medical treatment.

What It Is

The root of the word *prayer* comes from a Latin word that means "obtained by entreaty." In virtually all cultures there have been prayers for rites of passage through life, such as birth, adulthood, marriage, and death.

The application of prayer takes many forms. Prayers may be read silently or spoken aloud. Prayer also can be a silent form of meditation. Some prayers are improvised while others follow a set form. Praying may occur individually or in a group; it may focus on oneself or on helping others. **Intercessory prayers**, which are offered

Figure 33 For many, prayer is a powerful asset in times of illness and emotional need.

for others who are often geographically distant, have been the subject of recent investigation.

Many religions adhere to established times and rituals for organized prayer. Tibetan Buddhists construct prayer wheels, cylinders of wood and metal, with prayers written on them. Islam has five periods of prayer each day. In Western cultures, many parents teach their children to "say their prayers" at bedtime. The Catholic Church historically has divided the monastery day into seven segments and assigned particular psalms and prayers to each, such as matins and lauds, which comprise the morning prayers, and compline, the final canonical hour. Life in a monastery thus is a timed program of work, prayer, and rest.

What Practitioners Say It Does

The major health-related claim for prayer is that, even if it cannot effect cure, it can mitigate the adverse effects of disease, speed recovery, and increase the effectiveness of medical treatment.

Some groups, such as Christian Scientists, rely on prayer in lieu of conventional medical therapy, claiming that prayer alone can heal disease. Christian Science practitioners attribute illness to spiritual rather than organic causes. Most mainstream religious groups, however, do not reject conventional medicine. Indeed, the earliest European hospitals were developed and run by the Church, and many Christian and Jewish groups have founded, operated, and/or financially supported numerous American hospitals.

Beliefs on Which It Is Based

Across different religious traditions, explanations for the efficacy of prayer include a similar set of beliefs. These include the conviction that a deity or higher powers exist; that human beings can communicate with them through prayer; and that this God or gods can understand and act on human prayers, thereby influencing the course of illness.

Other explanations for the efficacy of prayer that do not rely on a specific deity have been advanced. For example, Larry Dossey, M.D., an author of popular books about healing and spirituality, developed a theory of "nonlocal medicine." The mind, he believes, is not limited to the physical brain. Instead, the minds of all people ultimately are joined, unbounded by space and time. This joining of consciousness, according to Dossey, allows prayer and other distance-healing methods to work by enabling the mind of one person to affect the mind—and therefore the health—of another. Dossey claims that nonlocal medicine cannot be explained in terms of current scientific knowledge because it postulates that the mind can transcend physical constraints such as time and location. This conceptualization of the mind and its powers is not consistent with contemporary science.

Research Evidence to Date

Studies of prayer and spirituality address several distinct types of activity. Research has examined the effects of intercessory prayer as well as the question of whether religious belief in and of itself can affect health.

There have been at least four published studies of intercessory prayer. Two double-blind studies, reported in the 1960s British medical literature, found no statistically significant effect for distant, intercessory prayer involving groups of people praying for patients. These studies were double-blind, meaning that neither the researcher nor the subjects knew which subjects were being prayed for. A recent study in New Mexico in which Jewish and Christian people prayed to relieve others' substance abuse problems found no effect for prayer.

The most famous study of intercessory prayer was conducted in the early 1980s at a coronary care unit in San Francisco—most famous because it is the only one that showed a benefit for intercessory prayer. In this study, 192 patients were prayed for by distant groups, while 201 patients with similar medical problems received no prayer. Prayers were directed at keeping these seriously ill patients alive. Results showed that prayed-for patients were less likely to require antibiotics and less likely to develop some complications, such as pulmonary edema.

However, there was no difference in mortality or length of stay in the coronary care unit between the two groups, although the prayers specifically asked to prevent death.

Restoring Health with External Energy Forces

In addition to that critical negative result, critics have pointed to major flaws in this study. For example, more than twenty-five medical variables were investigated, but differences between the prayed-for group and the control group occurred in only six of those variables. Furthermore, there is no way to control for or even know whether the control group really did not receive prayers from others, such as their friends and families.

From the perspective of serious theologians, these investigative approaches fail to test the effects of the real purpose of prayer, which is to earn the grace to draw from suffering whatever good is in it—to deal with the suffering and direct it into positive channels. This attitude itself may affect health. Praying to prevent death in oneself or others is not consistent with the true purpose of prayer from a theological view.

Another body of literature has attempted to determine whether religious belief confers a health benefit. Literature reviews of these studies reveal mixed results. In an analysis of 115 studies, thirty-seven studies found that religious belief seemed to have a positive effect on health, forty-seven studies produced a negative effect, and thirty-one found no effect. Another survey looked at religious involvement as an in-depth measure of religious practice. Twenty-two of twenty-seven studies showed regular religious involvement to have a positive effect on health. Such involvement could contribute by virtue of religiosity, social support, prayer, or some other mechanism.

Other recent studies also find benefits for religious activity. Work at Duke University Medical Center found that older patients involved in regular religious practices were less likely to be depressed than those who were not, including elderly patients with serious disabilities, a group statistically more prone than average to depression.

A widely reported study at Dartmouth found that, following open heart surgery, patients who had strong social support or who derived strength and comfort from their religion experienced lower mortality than those without such support or religious comfort. If they had *both* strong social support and religious belief, their risk of mortality was lowered even more dramatically.

Personal belief also has been shown to be an important component of the **relaxation response** (see Chapter 18). Researchers find that an important component of eliciting the relaxation response is repeating a word or very brief phrase with personal meaning. However, it is important to note that the content of the phrase does not matter; it is the meaning of the phrase to the meditator that is significant. The phrase, "The Lord is my shepherd" works for Christians, the word "shalom" works for Jews, Buddhists and others often prefer long vowel sounds, and words such as "love" or "one" or "peace" work for those without any particular religious belief.

The fact that religion and religious practices have existed in virtually every culture throughout history suggests to some scientists that an evolutionary survival advantage may be conferred by religious belief.

What It Can Do For You

Without attempting to contest individual religious belief, the scientific evidence suggests that intercessory prayer has not been proven to influence the course of illness, either in a positive or negative way.

As for the health benefits of religious belief, there are some studies that appear to indicate that religious belief does correlate with better health. However, it is important to note that correlation is not the same as causation; other factors, such as social support, may explain the better health of those with religious belief. The evidence is not yet clear that religious faith causes better health.

Whether or not prayer and spirituality confer direct health benefits, many people find religion to be an important part of their lives by providing meaning, fellowship, and comfort (Figure 33). Those benefits are themselves intrinsically helpful, stress-reducing, and consistent with good health practices.

Where to Get It

Prayer and spirituality are areas of individual conscience and personal belief. Some prefer praying in solitude, while others feel enriched by a community of people who share the same beliefs or by the presence and words of a spiritual leader. You are the best guide to developing your own spirituality and religious life.

Restoring Health with External Energy Forces

53

Shamanism

Shamans are religious leaders or priests believed by their community to have the ability to cure the sick through magical powers. Shamanic healing, which appeared in early cultures throughout most of the world, displays characteristics of both religion and magic, as did all early efforts to deal with illness and other undesirable events.

Perhaps the oldest of all healing therapies, shamanism originated over 20,000 years ago—some researchers say 40,000 —in the Altai and Ural Mountains of western China and Russia. The word *shaman* in the Tungusu-Manchurian language means "to know."

To his or her tribe, the shaman is the only person capable of communicating with ancestral spirits, gods, and demons, which remain invisible to others. It is through this unusual power that the shaman can divine the unseen, control events, and thereby cure disease.

Other early cultures, including those on the North and South American continents, in Asia, India, Africa, the South Pacific, and Australia, all had their own concepts of a shaman: religious leader, healer, and seer. Shamans used rituals that included singing, dancing, chanting, drumming, art forms, and storytelling to heal the sick, promote success in hunting and food gathering, and to create in other ways a safer or better life for members of their tribe.

In more modern times, especially among Native Americans (see Chapter 5), shamans add conventional medicine to their traditional practices to promote healing. At the same time, many shamans today share their knowledge about healing with others. This has encouraged a modern resurgence of interest in this oldest of healing therapies. Lectures, weekend meetings called "medicine wheel gatherings," and other group activities are now available to the general public. They teach shamanic principles such as living in balance with nature.

What It Is

Shamanism is a form of folk medicine, mind-body or

Powers and Responsibilities

Shamanism is a primitive religious system in which the shaman, or medicine man, is the central figure.

When in a trance state, the shaman is believed possessed by gods and spirits that act through him or her.

All powerful, the shaman is expected to restore health, protect the tribe, foretell the future, and otherwise guide and safeguard the community.

trance healing, or "white magic" that relies on healers with special powers. These healers, or shamans, mediate between hostile spiritual forces and the problems facing the people of their communities. Common problems include wounds and disease, childbirth, and overcoming evil spirits.

Most people around the world, although not in industrialized cultures, continue to rely on shamans or comparable healers for their health care (Figure 34). The "medicine man" often portrayed in old American cowboy and Indian movies was, in fact, a shaman, and Native Americans today call their shamans "medicine men." Shamans go through rigorous training before practicing their profession. They are often well paid by their patients, but also may suffer punishment if they fail to effect a cure.

The work of the shaman consists of more than the magic or religious rites typically conducted at night in locations with special religious significance. Throughout history, shamans also have discovered plants that have identifiable beneficial effects. These botanicals are applied to treat various ailments. However, contemporary shamans continue to blame ill-defined illnesses on spirits who must be placated before the patient can be cured.

In order to communicate with the spiritual world, the shaman goes into a trance or mind-altering process. This state is reached through fasting or the use of hallucinogenic herbs or plants, typically accompanied by chanting, drumming, and dancing. In the self-induced trance, the shaman's supernatural powers help him discover the cause of the illness or pain. He then seeks to intercede with evil spirits that caused the problem, thereby restoring his or her patient's health.

What Practitioners Say It Does

Shamans believe they have a special ability to communicate with the spiritual world through altered mental states. These states of ecstasy enable the shaman to journey to the unknown, communicate with spirits, gather knowledge, and return to reality to use that knowledge to heal the sick. The shaman's work promotes an expectation of recovery in the patient, who believes the battle with evil spirits will be won.

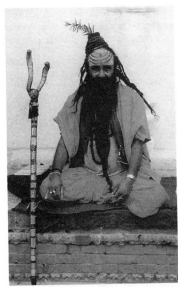

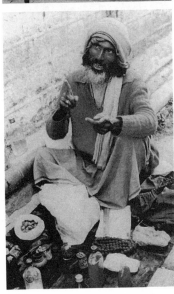

Figure 34 Across time, cultures, and continents, shamans, like these in Nepal today, offer charms, herbs, and ritual objects in addition to their magical healing skills.

Restoring Health with External Energy Forces

Shamanic therapy, including chanting, drumming, dancing, and spirit visualization, reportedly is used in a few clinics in the United States today.

Another contemporary activity, **psychic surgery**, is a modern expression of traditional Filipino shamanism. Practiced also in North America by visiting Filipino shamans, psychic surgery involves the extraction of "tumors" from the body through a bloody but painless and invisible "incision" in the patient's abdomen. Chicken blood and parts have been found hidden on the shamans who perform these procedures.

Whether shamans believe they can cure any and all diseases is not clear. It is interesting to note, however, that some shamans select their patients with care, feeling that their special talents will not be beneficial in every case. There is a fear of failure and its consequences of punishment by the tribe.

Beliefs on Which It Is Based

Shamanism is based on the belief that all healing has a spiritual dimension that must be addressed before healing can occur. It is believed that the evil spirits inhabiting the spiritual dimension contributed to the patient's sickness. It is further believed that the shaman, an individual with special training and the ability to enter into a self-induced trance, can communicate in that state of mental suspension with the spirit world. There the shaman has the opportunity to mediate with evil spirits on behalf of the patient, and perhaps gather knowledge on how best to cure the patient.

Research Evidence to Date

There is an abundance of historic material from many cultures and written over many centuries about the successes of shamanism and its ability to treat illness and other problems. This material consists of anecdotes, which are in essence stories similar to those attributed to religious miracles.

Shamanic practices have not been subjected to research as such. That is, studies have not been conducted to test the frequency or mechanisms of shamanic activity. However, expectation and strong belief are known to have powerful healing effects, as described in discussions of the placebo effect in Chapter 19 as well as in other chapters in this book.

At this time, there are no certification programs for shamans, nor is there a professional association representing them. The lack of both, in addition to the mystical quality of shamanic belief, may have discouraged scientific researchers from investigating the effectiveness of shamanic healing.

What It Can Do For You

A researcher and psychologist at Stanford University

in California reported that shamanistic practices sometimes are useful in treating pain, anxiety, and stress among cancer patients, especially Native American patients. The rhythmic drumming usually included in a shaman therapy session has been helpful in interrupting destructive thought patterns assumed to be detrimental to recovery from illness.

Many believe that shamanism can help promote spiritual or emotional healing. A therapeutic session with a shaman, or participation in a shamanic ritual with its chanting, drumming, and dancing, often produces outcomes similar to those effected by counselors or psychotherapists. Even if shamanic healing achieves its effect through a placebo-like response, that response can be comforting and beneficial to the patient.

Where to Get It

+ One of the best resources for information about modern shamanic activity is the Dance of the Deer Foundation (408 475-9560), an organization founded to promote continuation of the Huichol Indian shamanic tradition. The Foundation is located in Soquel, California, in the Santa Cruz Mountains. It promotes an active program of ongoing study groups, seminars, and pilgrimages throughout the world. Participants can learn practices of shamanic health and healing and how to live more balanced lives. The foundation has a home page on the Internet, and its e-mail address is shaman@shamanism.com.

+ The Foundation for Shamanic Studies in Mill Valley, California (415 380-8282), may also provide useful information. Those who visit or live near American Indian reservations also may learn more about shamanism by contacting tribal headquarters at each reservation.

54 ⌇

Therapeutic Touch

Therapeutic touch shares with other alternative and complementary therapies (such as *qigong*, tai chi, biofield therapies, Reiki, among others) belief in "energy fields" or "life forces" in and around the human body. There is no touch in therapeutic touch. Rather, the therapist's hands, held inches above the patient, sense and alter the hypothesized energy field around the patient's body.

Developed in the 1970s by Delores Krieger, Ph.D., R.N., then professor (and now Professor Emeritus) of nursing at New York University, with assistance from Dora Kunz, a clairvoyant, therapeutic touch has become very popular and is often practiced in hospitals, nursing homes, and other health-care facilities throughout the United States and elsewhere. Krieger estimates that she has taught the technique to more than 40,000 people as of 1995, and writes that her program is taught in over eighty U.S. universities and practiced in sixty-eight countries in addition to the United States.

Therapeutic touch is closely related to the concept of **laying on of hands**, practiced by ministers of several faiths and often used at revival meetings, during which healing energy is said to flow from the healer to the patient. The power of therapeutic touch, however, is derived not from a religious concept of God's presence, but rather from the idea of energy fields within and surrounding the body. "Energy field disturbances" is an official nursing diagnosis.

The value of touch is demonstrated in various therapies to provide a feeling of caring, security, and understanding between healer and patient. Historically, the idea is ancient; it can be identified in 15,000-year-old cave paintings found in the Pyrenees. It is important to note, however, that therapeutic touch, despite its name, does not include touching the person's body (Figure 35).

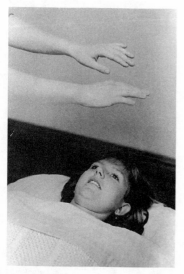

Figure 35 Therapeutic touch does not actually involve touching the physical body. Practitioners claim they are shifting the energy field that emanates from the patient's body.

What It Is

Practitioners hold their hands, palms down, a few inches above the patient's body. They sweep their hands from the patient's head to toe, shaking off the bad or excess energy after each sweep. Practitioners also transmit energy from their own hands to the patient's energy field.

A therapeutic touch session usually lasts for twenty to thirty minutes. The patient lies down, and the practitioner stands at the patient's side. Each session is divided into four activity segments:.

1. **Centering** The therapist focuses his or her own thoughts, clearing the mind to communicate with the patient's energy field and identify areas of abnormality or blockage of energy flow.

2. **Assessment** In this phase, the practitioner passes his or her hands, held two to six inches above the patient's body, down the length of the body, looking for blockages to the normal flow of energy. The therapist expects to be able to identify specific forces of emanating energy.

3. **Unruffling** To unruffle the patient's energy field and restore balance, the therapist sweeps stagnant energy downward past the patient's toes and out of the body.

4. **Transferring** The practitioner concludes the session by transferring his or her own excess energy to the patient, thereby altering any misalignment in the patient's energy field and relieving pain, curing illness, or accomplishing some other goal.

What Practitioners Say It Does

Proponents of therapeutic touch believe the human body produces its own energy field, and that blockages in the energy field cause illness and pain. Practitioners believe their hands can detect these blockages or imbalances. Advocates claim that practitioners can focus on the area causing pain, transfer their own energy, and change the patient's energy field, thereby stimulating the body's own recuperative powers.

Practitioners believe that therapeutic touch reduces stress and promotes relaxation, cures headaches, reduces anxiety, and stimulates a sick person's recuperative powers. It is also said to calm crying babies, alter enzyme activity, increase hemoglobin levels, reduce fever and inflammation, ease asthmatic breathing, and accelerate the healing of wounds.

Beliefs on Which It Is Based

Because there is no scientific evidence to show how or why it works, or even to support the existence of an energy field, therapeutic touch requires faith in the existence of such a field and in the ability of therapeutic touch to alter it. The basic belief is the presence of a life force or energy field, similar to *qi* in Chinese medicine and *prana* in Ayurvedic (ancient Indian) medicine.

Krieger says she was influenced by yoga, Ayurvedic, Tibetan, and Chinese health systems in developing these concepts. Her theories of energy transfer are based on the belief in energy fields that was essential to ancient Asian and Indian therapies. She points out that the concept of a life force or energy field around human bodies, although unproven, does not contradict the laws of modern physics, which state that all matter contains energy.

Krieger believes there may be a relationship between therapeutic touch and blood hemoglobin that distributes oxygen throughout the body. She believes that when touch therapists transfer energy to the patient, the energy increases the patient's hemoglobin levels, thereby enhancing the oxygen supply, which in turn increases vitality .

Although some practitioners are at a loss to understand how they can transfer energy from their own bodies to that of the patient, most are confident they are able to do so.

Research Evidence to Date

No objective, scientific studies about therapeutic touch have been published in reputable journals, but much has been written by Krieger and other nurses. In addition, an abundance of anecdotal reports describe its successes. Although widely employed by nurses, therapeutic touch nevertheless remains unexplained within the constraints of contemporary science.

What It Can Do For You

People who seek therapeutic touch tend to feel better after the experience. For some, it can assist relaxation, reduce stress, relieve headaches, and ameliorate the discomforts of illness, injury, and surgery. Regardless of

The Alternative Medicine Handbook

whether energy transfer does or does not exist, the sheer attention and the therapist's hands passing over the body no doubt enhance a sense of well-being.

Despite the need to take therapeutic touch on faith because there is no scientific evidence of its existence or effectiveness, hundreds of success stories report the alleviation of patients' various aches and pains. Scientists suggest that patients' reactions may reflect a kind of placebo response, or that psychological benefits may accrue simply from having a caring person nearby, providing concern and attention.

Where to Get It

+ As is true for most therapies, therapeutic touch resources are listed in the Yellow Pages of your telephone directory under the section labeled "Massage Therapists." Massage therapists who practice therapeutic touch usually so indicate in their advertising.
+ The therapeutic touch organization, Nurse Healers Professional Associates, Inc., is located at 175 Fifth Avenue, New York, NY 10010. The organization was founded by Dolores Krieger.
+ The American Massage Therapy Association in Evanston, Illinois (312 761-2682), although not specifically organized around therapeutic touch, maintains relevant information.

COMPLEMENTARY THERAPIES
FOR SOME COMMON AILMENTS

acne The herb arnica.

alcohol and drug abuse Acupuncture, meditation, mental imagery.

anemia, caused by iron deficiency Diet adjustments or nutritional supplements.

anxiety and stress Therapeutic massage, acupressure (press center of inside wrist 1 inch above crease), relaxation techniques, yoga, aromatherapy, tea made from dried valerian herb, high-quality Asian ginseng (animal data only).

arthritis Acupuncture, hand and back yoga exercises, hydrotherapy, dietary supplements glucosamine and chondroitin.

attention deficit disorder Biofeedback, B vitamin supplements.

backache Chiropractic, valerian, massage, and other bodywork.

bronchitis Zinc lozenges, inhale steam with oil of eucalyptus, drink elderberry tea.

burns (minor) Aloe gel, cream of arnica.

Carpel Tunnel Syndrome Hydrotherapy, massage, ginger compress.

cholesterol, high 1 to 5 cloves of fresh garlic or coated tablet with allicin yield of four grams of fresh garlic.

colds and flu Zinc lozenges, echinacea, eucalyptus or peppermint oil in steam vaporizer, salt gargle, elderberry tea, herbs that calm coughs: Iceland moss, plantain leaves, slippery elm, chew clove of raw garlic as antibiotic.

constipation Drink 6 to 8 glasses of water daily, eat more fiber, plantago seed, cascara, buckthorn bark, alfalfa sprouts and tablets.

depression Hypericum (St. John's wort), yoga, tai chi, meditation, light therapy.

diarrhea Dried blackberry, blueberry, or raspberry leaves, dried blueberry fruit, peppermint tea.

headache Press acupoints between eyebrows or in hollows at base of skull on both sides of spine, massage, progressive relaxation, biofeedback, feverfew capsules can prevent migraines.

heartburn Ginger tea.

high blood pressure Garlic, foods rich in calcium and magnesium, mind-body techniques.

impotence Relaxation techniques (ginkgo and ginseng are unproven).

indigestion Peppermint or chamomile tea.

menopause problems Black cohosh extracts, vitamin E.

menstrual cramps Warm baths, feverfew, extract of the herb black cohosh, raspberry leaf tea, yoga positions.

motion sickness/nausea Ginger (tea, capsules, candy), press acupoint at center of inside wrist, an inch above wrist crease.

muscle aches Volatile mustard oil, wintergreen oil, capsicum cream, massage, hydrotherapy.

osteoporosis Walking and other weight-bearing exercises, calcium-rich diet or supplements can help prevent or slow progression.

pain, chronic Acupuncture, massage and other body work, biofeedback, hypnotherapy.

PMS Lavender or parsley oil in a warm bath, yoga, meditation, black cohosh extract.

prostate enlargement Saw palmetto extract, nettle root tea.

rashes Soak oak bark or English walnut leaf in boiling water; when cool, apply to skin.

Seasonal Affective Disorder Depression therapies, especially light therapy.

sleep problems Valerian tea, warm bath, massage, meditation.

sunburn Bathe in cool water with baking soda, apply aloe gel, apply arnica cream.

tennis elbow Acupuncture, bodywork techniques, chiropractic, apply ice.

urinary tract infections Drink bearberry leaf–soaked cold water, cranberry juice.

varicose veins Horse chestnut seed ointment, yoga, elevate feet.

warts Hypnosis, apply dandelion juice.

GLOSSARY

acupoints Points or places along the body's meridians where needles or pressure are applied.

acupressure Hand or finger pressure applied to an acupuncture point on the body.

acupuncture Therapy using very thin needles inserted at designated points (acupoints) along meridians on the body to balance the hypothesized flow of energy and to restore health.

acute Having a short, sometimes severe course. Not chronic.

Alexander technique A type of movement therapy intended to reduce muscular tension. This technique is useful as a complementary therapy in treating stress, muscular fatigue, and neck and back pain.

allergen Any substance capable of producing an immediate hypersensitivity or allergy. Dust and pollen are typical allergens.

allopathic medicine Mainstream or modern medicine; based on principles proven through scientific research. Contrast with "alternative medicine."

alternative medicine Therapies used in place of allopathic medicine; not proven by traditional scientific investigation.

antioxidant A natural or synthetic substance, such as vitamin E, that prevents or delays the oxidation process in cells or tissue.

aromatherapy The therapeutic use of odors distilled from plant oils; said to be useful in treating headaches, anxiety, and tension.

art therapy The use of drawing, painting, and sculpting as therapy to treat behavior or emotional problems; promotes self-expression.

artery The vessels that circulate blood from the heart to various parts of the body.

aura An atmosphere said to surround a person. In alternative medicine, it is believed that everyone has a surrounding aura (energy field), visible to some people, that indicates the individual's state of health.

Ayurvedic medicine An ancient traditional medicine system based on Hindu philosophy and ancient Indian civilization. The human body is seen as a microcosm of the universe, consisting of the five elements of fire, water, earth, air, and ether. Each element corresponds to one of the five senses: sight, taste, smell, touch, and hearing. It embraces the concept of an energy force in the body similar to the Chinese concept of *qi* and emphasizes the balance of mind, body, and spirit to maintain health.

Bach flower remedies The use of oils from one or more of thirty-eight different flowers as self-treatment therapies for mental, emotional, and sometimes physical discomfort.

bacteria Single-cell microorganisms living in air, soil, and water and as parasites in the bodies of plants and animals. Some types cause disease in humans.

benign Nonthreatening to health or life; a noncancerous growth.

biofeedback The use of electrical devices to recognize changes in body functions (such as heart rate, perspiration, and temperature) to achieve relaxation or muscle control. Sometimes used to treat incontinence, stress, and anxiety-related conditions.

biopsy A diagnostic technique that examines tissues, fluids, or cells removed from the human body.

biorhythms Individual physical, mental, or emotional cycles, lasting typically twenty-two to thirty-three days; often charted by naturopathic physicians to better understand behavior and determine most opportune times for treating depression and illness.

bodywork A broad term used to identify a variety of techniques to promote relaxation through massage, manipulation, controlled movement, reflexology, and other hands-on procedures. It includes standard Swedish massage, the Alexander technique, the

Feldenkreis method, Rolfing, Hellerwork, and other variations.

botanical medicine Use of the entire plant or herb for therapeutic purposes.

capillaries The smallest blood vessels in the body. They connect to tiny arteries and veins.

carbohydrate The major class of foods that includes starches, sugars, cellulose, and gums. Carbohydrates are a necessary part of the daily diet.

carcinogen Any cancer-causing substance.

cartilage Dense, flexible connective tissue found at the ends of some bones, in the nose, and elsewhere in the body.

catheterization The process of inserting a catheter or small tubular device into a vessel, body cavity, or organ such as the bladder or heart in order to examine it with a tiny video camera, to inject or remove fluids, or to open passageways.

channels Passageways in the body through which the hypothesized life force identified as *qi* or *prana* is said to travel; also called meridians.

chemotherapy The use of chemicals that do not harm most normal tissue, but that attack fast growing cells such as cancer cells.

chi see "*qi*"

Chinese herbal medicine A mainstay of the 3,000-year-old Chinese system of comprehensive health and healing. Thousands of different herbs are used to treat specific complaints.

chiropractic The largest nonsurgical and drugless system of healing in the West. Chiropractic assumes that a smooth flow of nerve impulses from the brain to all parts of the body through the spinal column is necessary for maintaining homeostasis or equilibrium among different parts of the body, and thus good health. Misaligned vertebrae, called subluxations, are thought to interfere with the transmission of nerve impulses. The chiropractor uses manipulation to reposition spinal bones.

cholesterol A steroid alcohol found in animal cells and body fluids. The human liver usually produces sufficient cholesterol to meet bodily needs. Diets high in saturated fats usually increase cholesterol levels in the blood, creating an unhealthy condition that can lead to coronary heart disease.

chromatotherapy The unproven belief that colored lights can help cure serious diseases such as cancer.

chromosome A structure found in the nucleus of each human cell. It contains DNA, which transmits genetic information during cell division. There are typically forty-six chromosomes in each cell.

chronic Continuing over a long period of time; not acute.

collagen An insoluble protein found in skin, bone, cartilage, and other connective tissue.

colonic irrigation A form of hydrotherapy that uses large amounts of water to irrigate the large bowel. It is said to relieve constipation, detoxify the colon, and aid elimination.

colored-light therapy An unproven therapy that uses different colors of lights for therapeutic purposes. Some colors are believed to have a specific effect on specific diseases. Red light, for example, is believed to stimulate the sympathetic nervous system.

complementary medicine Medical care that is adjunctive (used in addition to) traditional medical care. Most complementary therapies are beneficial in promoting relaxation, reducing stress, and controlling symptoms.

counseling Professional guidance or direction provided through talk therapy.

cranial osteopathy A specialized diagnostic and therapeutic process based on reducing subtle movements of the bones of the skull through manipulation. Because the bones of the skull become fused in early childhood, this technique is improbable as well as unproven.

craniosacral therapy A manipulative therapy designed to treat the craniosacral system, including the cranium, sacrum, spinal cord, and bones of the spine; closely related to cranial osteopathy.

crystal healing Sometimes called gem therapy; uses quartz crystals and gemstones, which are believed to emit electromagnetic energy, for healing purposes; often used in combination with color therapy.

cupping An ancient Chinese and Ayurvedic therapy that aims to lower blood pressure, improve circulation, and relieve muscle pain by making punctures in the skin and then covering them with a heated cup which creates suction. Cupping was also used in colonial American medicine.

dehydration The loss of water from the body.

An abnormal and sometimes dangerous depletion of body fluids.

detoxification The process of removing "toxic substances" from the body; treatment to free an individual from a chemical addiction.

dietary therapy The use of diet, or prescribed food intake, to effect health benefits. Unproven or fad diets can be harmful because of severely imbalanced nutritional intake. Diets that claim to cure cancer and other diseases are fraudulent.

disease A condition that impairs the function of a person or body organ.

doshas The three basic body types or life forces that underlie human functioning according to Ayurvedic belief. They are *Veda*, producing movement; *Kapha*, responsible for bodily structure; and *Pitta*, an interface between *Veda* and *Kapha*.

electromagnetic therapy A form of "energy medicine" that claims to diagnose and correct disturbed electromagnetic frequencies emitted by the body, thus curing disease and promoting health. Many mysterious "black boxes" are marketed from time to time as electrical devices capable of producing cures. Although electric energy is used in many traditional diagnostic devices such as X rays and MRIs (magnetic resonance imaging), there is no evidence that electromagnetic therapy cures disease.

energy therapies A broad range of treatments based on the use of various energy forms to heal illness and disease. Electroacupuncture, electromagnetic therapy, dental energy medicine, microwave energy, and other approaches utilize a variety of electrical devices. The TENS (transcutaneous electrical nerve stimulator) unit is useful for reduction of pain. The use of highly charged electric paddles in a hospital emergency department to restart a stopped heart is also a common practice. Most others are unproven.

enzyme A complex protein that acts as a chemical catalyst between other substances without themselves being destroyed or altered. Enzymes are divided into six categories according to the work they do in the body, such as the conversion of proteins and sugars.

essential oil Highly concentrated aromatic oil used in aromatherapy. The forty different oils designed to treat specific ailments are derived from roots, bark, leaves, wood, and sap of plants, trees, and herbs. The rinds of citrus fruits also provide fragrant essential oils. Because of their highly concentrated aromas, they are usually diluted in "carrier" oils or alcoholic solutions.

etiology The cause or origin of disease.

extract A concentrated preparation such as an essence or concentrate created by withdrawing the active constituents by chemical or physical processes prepared as semiliquids, dry powders, or solids.

fasting Technically, abstention from eating. In alternative medicine, fasting purports to cleanse the body of impurities, based on the notion that when the body is not digesting food, greater reserves of energy are available for use in immune function, cell growth, and elimination processes. Because the body is deprived of necessary energy resources during fasting, it can be dangerous.

fat One of the three kinds of food energy, along with carbohydrates and proteins. Fats are found in meat, poultry, fish, dairy products, and some vegetables. The goverment's food pyramid guide recommends two to three servings of fat from meat, poultry, fish, and/or dairy products each day. Stored in the human body as adipose tissue, fat provides a major reserve source of energy. It also acts as a "padding" between various organs of the body. It protects against cold and helps the body absorb certain vitamins. Excess dietary fat increases the risk for serious health problems.

fatty acid A component of fat, whether saturated, monounsaturated, or polyunsaturated. Saturated fats raise blood cholesterol levels.

Feldenkrais method A therapy designed to make the body work with gravity rather than against it by correcting physical habits of movement that unduly strain muscles and joints.

fiber Indigestible parts of plants, some soluble, some insoluble. In the human digestive system, fiber absorbs water and assists elimination. It is an essential part of a healthy diet.

flower remedies See "Bach flower remedies."

food guide pyramid Pyramid-shaped display of optimal nutritional intake, developed by the U.S. Departments of Agriculture and Health and Human Services.

free radical An unstable molecule with an odd number of electrons, produced as a by-product of oxidation. Free radicals are potentially harmful to the body, as interaction with DNA can lead to impaired cell function, and they may be a factor in development of cancer. Said to be neutralized by antioxidants.

friction A type of massage employing small circular movements of the fingers and thumbs or the heel of the hand. One of six major massage techniques.

fungus A parasitic organism such as a mold or yeast that can infect human body tissue.

gene A segment of a DNA molecule and the biological unit of heredity. It is self-reproducing and transmitted from parent to progeny.

generic drug A medication without a specific brand name. After patent rights expire on brand-name medications, similar generic drugs are often produced and marketed at lower cost to the consumer.

Hellerwork An outgrowth of Rolfing, this bodywork therapy concentrates on efficient body movements seen as natural to different body types. Alignment with the earth's gravitational forces is believed paramount, as is greater mind-body awareness.

herb A plant or plant part valued for medicinal or other purposes. Culinary herbs are used as flavoring in cooking.

herbal medicine Healing through the use of organic substances. One of the oldest forms of medical care, the ancient Egyptians, Chinese, Indians, and other early societies discovered that certain plants had curative properties. Myth and science over time have produced a system of therapies that range from the Doctrine of Signatures, in which an herb bearing physical characteristics similar to those of the illness to be treated would provide curative values, to the present-day pharmaceutical industry that produces medications synthesized from herbs. Chinese and Ayuravedic shamans, Indian medicine men, and modern practitioners have all used a wide variety of herbs to promote cures.

homeopathy A system of medicine based on the concept of "like cures like" (the Law of Similars): symptoms are treated with minute amounts of drugs that would normally produce the same symptoms as the illness being treated. Homeopathy was developed by a German physician and chemist as an alternative to the more severe practices of bloodletting, vomiting, and other excesses of ortho-dox medicine practiced in the early 1800s.

homeostasis An internal state of stability toward which the body automatically strives.

hormone One of many chemicals produced in the body by glands and certain organs. Hormones regulate activities of body systems, glands, organs, and tissues, usually distant from their originating source. Hormones regulate blood sugar levels, women's menstrual cycles, and growth.

hydrotherapy The use of water (hot or cold liquid, ice, or steam) to maintain or restore health. Forms of hydrotherapy include full-body immersion, saunas and steam baths, sitz baths, colonic irrigation, jacuzzis, and the use of hot or cold compresses.

hypnotherapy The use of hypnosis to treat or manage certain medical and psychological problems; often used to treat stress, sleeping disorders, anxiety, fears and phobias, and depression; also used to assist smoking cessation and to overcome alcohol and substance abuse.

infection The invasion of microorganisms and their subsequent multiplication in body tissues. A localized infection can become systemic if infecting microorganisms gain access to the lymphatic or vascular system.

inflammation A protective response to injury or destruction of body tissue; a localized action to destroy or isolate injured tissue and the injurious agent.

ligament A band of fibrous tissue that connects bones and cartilages and strengthens and supports joints.

light therapy The use of light and color to treat a variety of health problems, from depression to cancer. Full-spectrum and bright white light are used to effectively treat seasonal affective disorder (SAD), but practitioners' claims for its ability to treat most other health problems remain unsubstantiated.

macrobiotic diet A system stressing a life balance between yin and yang qualities: yin foods grow above ground and usually have a high water content, while yang foods tend to be roots, stems and seeds grown in colder, wet environments. Grains are closest to a neutrality between yin and yang and are therefore the most important component of the macrobiotic diet. Utensils used to prepare foods are carefully chosen, avoiding copper or aluminum. Lengthy cooking is usually required. Malnutrition is a potential problem.

magnetic therapy See "electromagnetic therapy."

malignant Tending to metastasize and infiltrate. Used in describing cancerous tissue or tumors of potentially unlimited growth.

mammography Low-dose X rays of the breast to detect abnormalities such as cancer.

mantra An uplifting, sometimes mystical word or phrase usually associated with meditation. In Ayurvedic medicine, a category of Satvajaya, or sound therapy, designed to change the vibratory patterns of the mind.

massage Manipulation of tissues and muscles by rubbing, stroking, kneading, or tapping. It is the most basic of all bodywork, frequently used for musculoskeletal problems.

meditation The process of focusing one's thoughts or engaging in contemplation or reflection. As a complementary therapy, a method of reaching the mind's inner reservoir of creative thought and energy, as in Transcendental Meditation. Meditation can lower heart rate and address some blood pressure problems, help alleviate chronic pain, and reduce stress.

megavitamin therapy Taking doses of vitamins far above levels recommended for general good health in order to prevent or cure certain diseases. Excessive amounts of certain vitamins can cause liver, bone, and nerve function damage as well as rapid pulse, insomnia, and other disorders.

meridians From ancient Chinese medicine, particularly acupuncture, the fourteen main channels of energy or life force that run up and down the body and head. Each meridian is said to affect a particular organ or body system.

metabolism Collectively, all of the physical and chemical processes through which life is sustained. Metabolic processes are fueled by energy from nutrients in food.

mineral An inorganic substance, neither animal or vegetable. Minerals are found in the human body in small amounts and are replenished from food. Naturally occurring springs, sometimes the center of health resorts, are often rich in minerals such as sodium, potassium, sulphur, or calcium.

moxa Another name for dried mugwort. Used in moxibustion by burning on the ends of needles, or rolled into sticks or cones that are then heated; said to increase the flow of *qi* in the body.

moxibustion (or moxabustion) A therapy used by Chinese herbal practitioners in which mugwort is burned on or very close to the body at an identified affected site to increase circulation and promote healing.

naturopathy (naturopathic medicine) A drugless therapy based on the body's own ability to heal itself, facilitated by a naturopathic physician trained to treat the cause rather than the effect of illness or disease. Treatments most often are diet- and nutrition-oriented with attention given to the patient's personal history and lifestyle.

needling The primary action of acupuncture. Very thin needles are inserted into the skin at key points along one of the many meridians or life-force lines on the body said to change the energy flow and thus promote healing.

nutritional therapy The use of dietary strategies to promote good health or treat illness.

orthodox medicine Health care based on scientifically proven principles; conventional medical care, practiced by physicians trained in recognized medical schools. The dominant type of care practiced in most developed nations in the world.

orthomolecular therapy See "megavitamin therapy"

osteopathy A medical philosophy based on the concept that the body can fight disease if it is in a "normal structural relationship," is adequately nourished, and is not adversely affected by environmental conditions. It follows generally accepted physical, surgical, and medicinal techniques for treatment and diagnosis. Some osteopathic physicians practice joint manipulation, postural reeducation, and physical therapy to correct structural problems.

OTC (over the counter) Describes medications legally sold without a physician's prescription. Many cold remedies, aspirin, Tylenol, and products for indigestion are OTC medications.

placebo effect Healing that results from the patient's belief in the treatment or therapist.

polarity therapy Based on the concept that in health, life energy circulates within and around the body in five specific patterns of dynamic balance, similar to the five environmental elements of Ayurvedic medicine. One of these elements of energy flows through each finger and toe. When the normal energy pattern is interrupted, gentle manipulative therapy is applied to eliminate blockages, restore balance, and promote relaxation. Yoga exercises, diet, and counseling also are applied.

prana Ancient Indian concept of healing energy or "force," equivalent to traditional Chinese medicine's *qi*.

progesterone A female sex hormone, secreted by the ovaries, that prepares the uterus for the reception and development of fertilized eggs. Along with estrogen, it regulates menstrual-cycle changes.

protein The primary and essential constituent of the protoplasm of all cells, consisting of complex combinations of amino acids. Protein, along with carbohydrates and fats, make up the three primary dietary components. Meat, fish, poultry, eggs, and dried beans are major sources of protein.

proving In homeopathy, testing a remedy by seeing what symptoms it elicits in healthy people.

psychosomatic Concerned with relationship between mind and body. Some bodily symptoms may be caused by mental or emotional disturbances, and are called psychosomatic.

qi According to ancient Chinese philosophy, the vital life "force" or energy that flows throughout the body along pathways that connect all organs and systems. Disruptions in the flow of *qi* (pronounced "chee"; also spelled *chi*) is said to cause imbalance and illness. Acupuncture is used to adjust *qi*.

qigong Traditional Chinese medicine regimen involving movements, breath regulation, and meditation, geared to balance *qi* and maintain health.

radionics A "black box" approach to diagnosis (or analysis) and holistic treatment; banned in the United States. "Corrective" energy patterns are directed from the instrument to the patient, even at a distance, to treat deep-seated health problems. The devices often analyze samplings from the patient, such as a snippet of hair, to arrive at a diagnosis.

RDA (Recommended Dietary, or Daily, Allowance) Guidelines developed by the Food and Nutrition Board of the National Research Council setting recommended levels of vitamins and minerals generally essential to good health. Figures published on processed food packaging as "Nutrition Facts" are based on a person requiring a 2,000-calorie-per-day diet.

red blood cell Blood cells that contain the protein hemoglobin, which carries oxygen from the lungs to the body. A shortage of these cells causes anemia.

reflexology A therapy that involves manipulation of the feet to promote homeostasis (balance) among body systems. Reflexologists believe that parts of the feet (reflex points) are related to specific body organs or functions. Stimulation by finger and thumb massage is believed to eliminate energy blockages that cause health problems.

relaxation response Decreased metabolism and other calming physiological reactions to meditation; the body's stress-reducing regulation of internal activity.

relaxation therapies Therapies that release physical and mental tension; often included in broader therapeutic programs. Flotation therapy, hypnotherapy, meditation, yoga, and many other mind-body therapies embrace relaxation-therapy principles.

remission A condition during which symptoms of a disease diminish or subside.

Rolfing A deep-tissue massage therapy, also called Structural Integration, designed to reach the body's connective tissue or fascias. Its intent is to strength and realign the body by stretching and lengthening the fascia. A treatment program usually consists of ten sessions which deal with different fascial layers sequentially. The therapist uses fingertips, knuckles, elbows, and sometimes knees to knead muscle and tissue layers.

Rosen technique A bodywork technique that treats the mind and body as one, believing that chronic muscle tension is caused by repressed emotional conflicts. Gentle, deep pressure is applied as the practitioner questions the patient about what he or she is experiencing.

seasonal affective disorder (SAD) Depression associated with the dwindling sunlight that occurs in winter. Geographic location plays a major role: people living in Canada or northern United States states are eight times more likely to experience SAD than are Southerners.

sedative An agent or drug that calms or moderates nervousness or excitement.

self-limiting Describes a condition that lasts a specific period of time and corrects or cures itself.

serotonin a brain neurotransmitter which at high levels can lead to relaxation and sleepiness; also a powerful vasoconstrictor (an agent that narrows the blood vessels).

shamanism A healing approach that dates back at least 20,000 years and found in almost every culture. The ability of shamans to enter a trance or a state of altered consciousness enables them to enter the spirit world, where they attempt to control the spirits and effect changes in the physical world. While in a trance, they believe their souls are separated from their bodies and transported throughout the cosmos in search of cures for their patients.

shiatsu Means "finger pressure" in Japanese; an Asian bodywork or acupressure technique in which fingers at specific points apply a firm sequence of rhythmic pressure to "awaken" acupuncture meridians.

Simonton method The use of imagery along with cancer therapy. Patients imagine their white cells as aggressive destroyers of their cancer cells.

sitz bath A form of hydrotherapy involving shallow, therapeutic immersion of the thighs and hips in warm water, sometimes with an additional substance in the solution such as Epsom salts; used as a tonic and to treat hemorrhoids and abdominal and pelvic disorders.

soft tissues Tissues of the body other than bone or cartilage; includes organs, muscles, tendons, and ligaments.

sound therapy An ancient method of healing based on the idea that everything in the universe, including the human body, is in a constant state of vibration and that even the slightest change in vibration can affect internal organs. It is believed that there is a natural frequency or note for each body part or organ, and that sound directed to a specific target can restore health to a body part whose vibration is out of kilter.

spiritual healing The transfer of a healing energy or life force from healer to patient through the laying on of hands. Some healers believe they have a God-given gift of healing or are helped by angels in their ability to channel cosmic energy from their hands to the patient.

Structural Integration see "Rolfing"

subluxations The term used by chiropractors to describe misalignments of the vertebrae; partial dislocations of bones in a joint.

supplement Something added; for example, food supplements taken in addition to meals. Complementary therapies used in addition to orthodox medicine can be termed supplemental therapies.

Swedish massage The most common form of massage, involving long gliding strokes, kneading, and friction on the superficial muscle layers; relieves muscle tension and promotes relaxation.

symptom Evidence of disease; something that suggests the presence of a bodily disorder.

syndrome A group of symptoms that occur together to produce a specific abnormality.

systemic Relating to or affecting the body generally.

tai chi An ancient Chinese system of gentle exercise or precision movement and breathing that develops balance, control, and relaxation and has calming effects. There are many specific sequences of movement in both long and short forms. Tai chi is used in treating stress-related problems and for rehabilitation after surgery, injury, and illness.

tendon The fibrous cord attached to muscles. It connects to other body parts.

TENS (transcutaneous electrical nerve stimulation) An electric device often used to treat affected nerves to relieve pain; accepted in mainstream medicine as a useful treatment for some diagnoses involving pain associated with the nervous system.

therapeutic touch A method of healing that does not include physical contact and so is not a true "touch" therapy, but rather one that deals with energy forces and the therapist's ability to transfer energy from his or her own body to that of the patient. The hands of the therapist pass inches above the patient's body, from head to toe in a wavelike motion, ending at the feet with a flick of the hands to dislodge any harmful energy.

tincture An alcohol or alcohol-and-water solution prepared from animal- or vegetable-based drugs.

toxin A poisonous substance produced by the metabolic activities of a living organism. Toxins are usually capable of inducing antibody formation in the body.

traditional Chinese medicine A complex healing system based on thousands of years of practice in the healing arts.

Trager approach A bodywork therapy in which gentle, rhythmic touch combined with movement exercises is applied by a therapist to release tensions in posture and movement in a procedure defined as Psychophysical Integration. It is a system of movement reeducation.

Transcendental Meditation (TM) Based on the Vedanta philosophy in Hinduism; a form of meditation that uses mantras (words or short phrases repeated in the mind) to exclude extraneous thought and reach a deep level of consciousness.

ultrasound High-frequency sound waves used to visualize internal organs for diagnostic purposes. In alternative medicine, ultrasound is used therapeutically to cause an increase in body temperature.

Vata One of the three basic forces and body types of Ayurvedic medicine. Symbolized by air, *Vata* is the *dosha* that produces movement.

vein The vessels through which blood low in oxygen passes from various body parts or organs back to the heart.

vertebrae Thirty-three bones of the spinal column. In chiropractic medicine, vertebrae out of alignment are believed to be the source of medical problems and are manipulated by the practitioner to restore health.

viruses Minute infectious agents capable of reproducing only in living host cells. Viral diseases include the common cold, influenza, mononucleosis, and AIDS.

visualization A relaxation therapy based on the formation of meaningful images in the mind. Mental pictures are used to achieve relaxation, reduce heart rate, and heal illness.

vitamins Organic substances in minute quantities that are vital to nutrition and good health. They help regulate body processes, but do not provide energy. Found in natural foods and sometimes produced by the body. Identified by letters and letter-number combinations (such as A, B, B_2) and sometimes by their chemical names (such as niacin and pantothenic acid).

white blood cells The primary resource in the immune system, the body's defense mechanism against disease. White blood cells attach themselves to infectious microbes and usually produce antibodies to destroy the invaders.

X ray A diagnostic device that uses electromagnetic radiation of a certain high frequency to create images used by radiologists to inspect and diagnose problems of the skeletal structure (especially bone fractures), potential cancerous sites, and other problems.

yin/yang Complementary but opposing qualities assigned to everything in the natural world as part of ancient Chinese cosmology. Everything has a yin and a corresponding yang as in night and day, hot and cold. The human body has both yin and yang organs which must produce a balance by operating in pairs. A balance of yin and yang forces in the body is assumed to create good health; when yin and yang are not balanced, illness results.

yoga An ancient Eastern philosophy of health and well-being. It is also a philosophy and exercise system that combines movement and simple poses with deep breathing and meditation to unite the human soul with a universal spirit. *Prana,* a life energy, is believed to flow through and vitalize the body. Those who practice yoga strive for a deep meditative state that promotes relaxation and reduces stress. It is a gentle exercise regimen suited to virtually any age group. Practiced as early as 3000 B.C.

PROFESSIONAL DEGREES
AND TITLES

B.M. Bachelor of Medicine

B.M.T Bachelor of Medical Technology

B.N. Bachelor of Nursing

B.S.N. Bachelor of Science in Nursing

C.A. Certified Acupuncturist

C.C.H. Certificate in Classical Homeopathy

C.M.A. Certified Medical Assistant

C.N.C. Certified Nutrition Consultant

C.N.M. Certified Nurse Midwife

D.C. Doctor of Chiropractic

D. Div. Doctor of Divinity

D.D.S. Doctor of Dental Surgery

D.H.A.N.P. Diplomate of Homeopathic Academy of Naturopathic Physicians

D.Ht. Doctor of Homeotherapeutics

D.I.B.A.K. Diplomate of the International Board of Applied Kinesiology

Dipl.Ac. Diplomate of Acupuncture

Dipl.C.H. Diplomate of Chinese Herbology

D.M.D. Doctor of Dental Medicine

D.O. Doctor of Osteopathy

D.O.M. Doctor of Oriental Medicine

D.P.E. Doctor of Physical Education

D.P.M. Doctor of Podiatric Medicine

D.Sc. Doctor of Sciences

D.S.W. Doctor of Social Welfare

D.Th. Doctor of Theology

D.T. Dietetic Technician

D.V.M. Doctor of Veterinary Medicine

F.I.C.C. Fellow of the International College of Chiropractors

F. N.A.A.O.M. Fellow of the National Academy of Acupuncture and Oriental Medicine

L.Ac. Licensed Acupuncturist

L.C.S.W. Licensed Clinical Social Worker

L.H.P. Licensed Homeopathic Physician

L.M.T. Licensed Massage Therapist

M.B. Bachelor of Medicine

M.D. Doctor of Medicine

M.D.(H.) Doctor of Homeopathic Medicine

M.Div. Master of Divinity

M.N.I.M.H. Master of the National Institutes of Medical Herbalists (British)

M.H. Master Herbalist

M.P.H. Master of Public Health

M.S.N. Master of Science in Nursing

M.S.P.H. Master of Science in Public Health

M.S.W. Master of Social Work

N.C.C.A. National Commission for the Certification of Acupuncturists

N.C.T.M.B. National Certificate in Therapeutic Massage and Bodywork

N.D. Doctor of Naturology (British); Doctor of Naturopathy (U.S.)

O.M.D. Oriental Medical Doctor

P.A. Physician's Assistant

Ph.D. Doctor of Philosophy

P.T. Physical Therapist

R.D. Registered Dietitian

R.N. Registered Nurse

R.Ph. Registered Pharmacist

INDEX

Burzynski, Stanislaw, 159–60
Byers, Dwight, 237, 239

cachexia, 162–63
Caisse, Renée, 162
calcium, 70, 75
Cancell, 160–61
cancer, 4–5, 33, 36, 49, 50, 51, 56,
    58, 66, 67, 68, 70, 86, 89, 97,
    99, 101, 102, 106, 113–14, 115,
    125, 128, 130, 132, 135, 137,
    141, 146, 151, 162–63, 234,
    250, 255, 257, 273, 306, 307–8
  alternative biological treatments
    for, 159–66
  breast, 5, 101, 102, 132, 223,
    277
  colon, 106, 277
  cures for, 63
  rectal, 277
capsicum cream, 92
carbon monoxide poisoning, 196
cardiac problems, see heart diease
carpal tunnel syndrome, 218, 229
cascara, 92
cat's claw (una de gata), 97
cayenne, 92
celiac disease, 183
cell therapy, 153, 154, 172–75
cellulase, 184
centaury, 84
centering, 319
cerato, 84
cerebral palsy, 302
cerebrospinal fluid, 222, 223
chakras, 25, 295–96
chamomile, 92, 259
Chan su, 97
chanting, 256
Chaparral tea, 97
Chase, Marian, 269
chelation therapy, 152–53, 154,
    176–78
chemotherapy, 56
  Revici's guided, 164–65
cherry plum, 84
chi (ch'i), 18–20
chicory, 84
childbirth, 49, 50, 61, 85, 125, 283,
    315
children, 104, 268
Chinese medicine, 6, 14, 15, 16–
    21, 22, 28–34, 39, 41, 58, 99,
    111, 145–48, 205, 207, 208,
    210, 236, 238, 243–47, 259,
    295, 320

Chinese mugwort (Artemisia vul-
    garis), 29
chiropractic, 203, 204–5, 206, 217–
    21, 222, 304
chloride, 75
cholesterol, 101, 102, 165
  LDL, 106
Christian Science Church, 305,
    309, 310
chromatotherapy, see light therapy
chromium, 75
chronic pain, 136, 151, 155, 192,
    214, 223, 281, 302
chronobiology, 276
cinnamon, 92
circadian rhythm, 276
cobalamin (vitamin B_{12}), 74, 104
coffee, 68, 180–81
coffee enemas, 58, 186, 187–88
cold–based hydrotherapies, 228–29
cold laser surgery, 167, 168
colds, 36, 39, 69, 89, 230, 233, 260
colon cancer, 106, 277
colon/detoxification therapies,
    152, 179–82
colonic irrigation, 186, 226, 228,
    231
coltsfoot, 97
communal healing, 44–45
constipation, 89, 146, 179, 233
Contreras, Ernesto, 186
Copeland, Royal, 38
copper, 75
coronary artery disease, 5, 106, 176
  see also heart disease
cortisol, 275
counseling, 48
Cousins, Norman, 272, 275
cranberries, 92
craniosacral therapy, 205, 222–25
crystal healing, 6, 291–92, 295–98
Cullen, William, 36
cupping, 17, 29–30, 32
cymatic therapy, 286, 287, 288
cystic fibrosis, 183
cystitis, interstitial, 161
cytosine arabinoside, 89

dance therapy, 256, 267–71
dandelion, 92–93
deafness, 269, 270, 282–83, 306
dentistry, biological, 153, 167–71
Depoloray, 300
depression, 5, 66, 85, 114, 137,
    147, 179, 233, 259, 273, 276,
    281, 312

DES, 61
detoxification, 187
devas, 297
diabetes, 36, 83, 86, 111, 114, 197,
    230, 233, 250, 302
diarrhea, 35, 39, 89
dietary supplements, 65–78, 186
diets, dietary remedies, 26, 48, 51,
    53–107
  regulation of, 60–64
  single food, 57
digestive-tract discomfort, 141
digitalis, 87
distress, 265
DMSO (dimethyl sulfoxide), 161
Doctrine of Signatures, 86
doshas, 24–27
Dossey, Larry, 310–11
double-blind studies, 140–41
Down's syndrome, 173, 174
drug abuse, see addiction

ear, electronic, 286
Ears Education and Retraining
    System (EERS), 286–87
eating disorders, 268
echinacea, 93
EDTA (ethylene diamine
    tetraacetic acid), 153, 176–78
effleurage, 232
elderberries, 93
elderly, 68, 269, 273, 312
electroacupuncture, 17
electrocardiogram (EKG; ECG),
    300
electroconvulsive therapy, 302
electrodermal activity (EDA), 118
electro-encephalogram (EEG), 300
electrogalvanism, 169–70
electromagnetic therapies, 292,
    299–304
electromyography (EMG), 117
electronic ear, 286
Electron-O-Ray, 300
Elixir Sulfanilamide, 61, 62
Ellis Micro-Dynameter, 301
Ellon USA, 85
elm, 84
endorphins, 211, 274, 275
enemas, 181–82
  coffee, 58, 186, 187–88
  shark cartilage, 198
energy flow, 205
English walnut leaves, 93
entrainment, 282
enzyme therapy, 153, 183–85

trepanation, 14
trigger points, 207
tuberculosis, 111, 306
tuina, 30

ulcers, 80, 111, 184, 302
ultrasound, 256, 286
ultraviolet light therapy, 276, 277
unruffling, 319
unsaturated fat, 106
Upledger, John, 222, 224
urinary incontinence, 120

valerian, 96
vascular disease, 230
Vata, 24–27
Vedas, 22
vegans, 104
vegetarianism, 56, 104–7
venom immunotherapy, 155–58
vetivert, 259
vibration, 232
vinca rosea, 86
vine, 84
viral illnesses, 184
vision quests, 44, 45
visual art therapy, 263–66

visual images, 23
visualization techniques, 127–30
vitamin A, 68, 71
vitamin B_1 (thiamine), 72
vitamin B_2 (riboflavin), 72
vitamin B_3 (niacin), 67, 72
vitamin B_5 (pantothenic acid), 65, 73
vitamin B_6 (pyrodoxine), 73
vitamin B_7 (biotin), 65, 73
vitamin B_9 (folic acid; folate), 68, 69, 73, 168
vitamin B_{12} (cobalamin), 74, 104
vitamin C (ascorbic acid), 58, 67, 68, 69, 70, 74, 168
vitamin D, 65, 68, 71, 104, 276, 278, 279
vitamin E, 68, 70, 71, 168
vitamin K, 71–72
vitamins, 55–78, 186
volatile mustard oil, 96
vomiting, 35
  induced, 26, 42
voodoo death, 141

walnut, 84
Warburg, Otto, 195

warts, 123
watercress, 96
water-soluble vitamins, 72–74
water violet, 84
whirlpool baths, 227
white-coat hypertension, 112
white sound, 285
wild rose, 84
willow, 84
willow tea, 42
Wilshire, Gaylord, 299–300
wintergreen oil, 96
witch hazel, 96–97

X rays, 303

Yellow Emperor's Classic of Internal Medicine, The, 232
yew tree, 90
yin-yang principle, 18–20, 28, 31, 99, 101, 245
yoga, 23, 26, 114, 120, 203, 204–5, 240, 248–51, 320
yohimbe bark, 97
Yuwipi, 43

zinc, 65, 69, 78